D1497823

"This book is a fantastic combination of an interesting read and a resource of life-changing information. I love the depth of knowledge and encouragement, and found myself making copious notes while reading chapter after chapter. It's a must-have for anyone interested in living a better, healthier, and more peaceful life."

—Dr. Georgina Cannon, award-winning author,
international expert on hypnosis and the mind-body connection

"As Dr. Mincolla points out, 'Here in the West, the very essence of life is rooted in materialism.' While there are many undesirable consequences of living in a materialistic age, one of the most significant is having lost sight of the miraculous, of which our own existence and all of life qualifies as such. As is pointed out in his book, the key to overcoming materialism and restoring our capacity to know the miraculous is to simply turn back to the spiritual, to the superconsciousness, to awareness itself our very own nature."

—Paul J. Mills, professor and chief of Family Medicine and
Public Health, University of California, San Diego

"In *The Way of Miracles*, Mark Mincolla describes how we can increase the probability that we will achieve desired outcomes and even generate miracles. He explains that we can do this by changing our guiding star to be our inner connection to Source instead of information in our external world and our ego consciousness. Offering stories of his and his patients' experiences—and information about neurobiology research, states of consciousness, nutrition, and practices of various spiritual traditions—he has made this an eminently useful and interesting book for anyone seeking tools for transformation."

—Carl Greer, PhD, PsyD, author of the award-winning bestseller
Change Your Story, Change Your Life

"*The Way of Miracles* focuses on a number of fundamental aspects of human life and explores the many possibilities available to all of us. Health and healing are often approached as goals to achieve in an external universe. However, both wisdom traditions and modern science seek wholeness in many similar ways. These can provide modern medicine with novel ways and tools to benefit humans. Modern quantum mechanics, like the ancient philosophical schools, places great emphasis on the role of the mind and how it interacts with what is perceived as an external cosmos. An evolving, yet eternal reality of Existence, in the field of what is certain and what is possible, all direct us to understand that complementarity, universality, and interactivity underlie our very lives. As such, the miracles that Dr. Mark Mincolla brings forth from his own professional experience may be quite common in health and healing, allowing ancient and modern views of Consciousness the central emphasis which can indeed change us in profound, in miraculous ways."

—Menas C. Kafatos, Fletcher Jones Endowed Chair Professor
of Computational Physics, Chapman University

"Mark Mincolla's *The Way of Miracles* sets the stage for you to create your own miracles. Leaving nothing to chance, he starts with his own journey to wholeness pulling you into this page turner. You will mark up and re-read, as you shift and evolve into your own wholeness, ultimately leading you to open the creative force within you. This is the key to unleash the power of miracles in you. An inspiring read it will expand your consciousness, making you a miracle worker, whether you believe it or not!"

—Maureen St. Germain, author of bestsellers *Waking Up in 5D*,
Opening the Akashic Records, and *Beyond the Flower of Life*

"*The Way of Miracles* is a lucid exploration of the fundamental state of all existence as pure consciousness in a field of infinite possibilities. This state of wholeness is also the basis of all healing. When we are whole, we are holy and healed. Mark Mincolla's personal journey of healing, and his understanding of states of consciousness as the basis of all experience, is profound. This book should convince you that life and existence are miracles and healing is a return to our original state of truth, awareness, and bliss."

—Deepak Chopra™, MD, bestselling author of *Metahuman*

THE WAY OF
MIRACLES

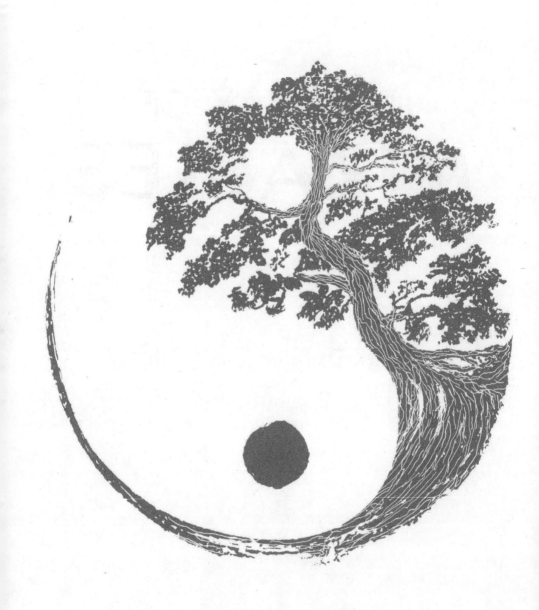

THE WAY OF
MIRACLES

Accessing Your Superconsciousness

MARK D. MINCOLLA, PhD

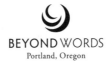

BEYOND WORDS
Portland, Oregon

BEYOND WORDS

1750 S.W. Skyline Blvd., Suite 20
Portland, OR 97221-2543
503-531-8700 / 503-531-8773 fax
www.beyondword.com

First Beyond Words hardcover edition June 2021

BEYOND WORDS PUBLISHING and colophon are registered trademarks of Beyond Words Publishing. Beyond Words is an imprint of Simon & Schuster, Inc.

For more information about special discounts for bulk purchases, please contact Beyond Words Special Sales at 503-531-8700 or specialsales@beyondword.com.

Managing Editor: Lindsay S. Easterbrooks-Brown
Editor: Brit Elders
Copyeditor: Kristin Thiel
Proofreader: Madison Schultz
Illustrations: Monique Miller-McCarthy
Design: Sara E. Blum
Composition: William H. Brunson Typography Services

Manufactured in the United States of America

10 9 8 7 6 5 4 3 2 1

Library of Congress Cataloging-in-Publication Data:

Names: Mincolla, Mark Dana, author.
Title: The way of miracles : accessing your superconsciousness / Mark D.
  Mincolla, Phd.
Description: First Beyond Words hardcover edition. | Portland, Oregon :
  Beyond Words, 2021. | Includes bibliographical references. | Summary:
  "The Way of Miracles is an adventure for the mind and spirit that begins
  with the premise that miracles don't randomly happen-we create them! "
  — Provided by publisher.
Identifiers: LCCN 2021003384 (print) | LCCN 2021003385 (ebook) | ISBN
  9781582708287 (hardcover) | ISBN 9781582708294 (ebook)
Subjects: LCSH: Holistic medicine. | Alternative medicine. | Mind and body
  therapies.
Classification: LCC R733 .M438 2021 (print) | LCC R733 (ebook) | DDC
  613—dc23
LC record available at https://lccn.loc.gov/2021003384
LC ebook record available at https://lccn.loc.gov/2021003385

The corporate mission of Beyond Words Publishing, Inc.: *Inspire to Integrity*

This book is dedicated to Fabiola Roht,
who inspired me and supported me every step of the way.

Our Source is boundless. It is part
of the infinite Universal field of
superconsciousness. It is a field that is
unlimited, and it is where miracles are
bountiful!

—Mark Mincolla, PhD

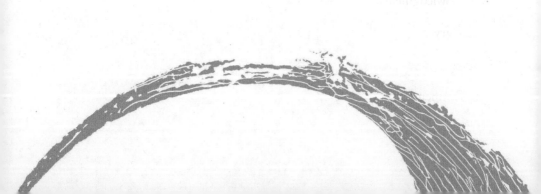

Contents

Foreword

This book has provided a greater appreciation of how miracles occur and how we, as individuals, are responsible for bringing them to fruition. I immediately related to Mark's understanding of how a person makes miracles in their life; I've personally experienced them, as you probably have. When miracles happen, we don't always recognize them because we haven't been instructed about the roles they play in our lives. Our analytical mind tends to set them aside as a moment of no consequence, when, in fact, the smallest miracle can be life altering. Mark provides methods and lessons for moving beyond the limited concept of nonacceptance to an all-encompassing cognitive awareness that *can* manifest miracles.

It's not difficult to achieve miracle-making possibilities, but it does require more than intent. The pathway to making miracles includes expectation, learning to follow or think with one's heart, and ultimately living in superconscious energy. Training the conscious mind to exist without fear, to broaden its perspective of the reality in which we exist, which includes all of the unseen energetic realities, and to be receptive to the limitless power of the Source prepares the way for healing and regenerative miracles that can truly affect one's life.

—*Brit Elders, CEO of ShirleyMacLaine.com*

Introduction

When I look around me, I see a world increasingly overcome with dis-ease and a healthcare industry that is increasingly out of touch with the deeper healing needs of the people it struggles to serve. It treats symptoms instead of substance and rarely exposes the fact that we need to heal, to be whole, on many different levels of our being. Because of this, I feel it's important to share a blueprint for optimum healing and health that I have utilized with tremendous success.

I'm a healer, a practitioner of natural, nutritional medicine. I've performed over sixty thousand consultations during the past thirty-seven years and feel blessed to have been a part of an unprecedented number of miracle healings during that time. Other physicians labeled most of these healing transformations hopeless, yet, miraculously, they happened.

The question is, Why did impossible recoveries happen?

While there's no question that personalized nutritional therapy contributed to the restoration of health, I realized that these miracles happened because of something beyond superfoods, special diets, and nutritional supplements. There was a very different kind of action present, an action that took both the patient and me, the practitioner, to another level.

The difference is superconsciousness, an energy that knows no boundaries. It's achieved by merging personal consciousness, or omnipresent awareness, that we are with that of the Universal mind.

By elevating the level of our awareness, we can access and attain the unlimited power of our whole being, and every one of us can create miracles that heal and inspire our lives. *The Way of Miracles: Accessing Your Superconsciousness* is a tool to help everyone connect to this ultimate healing power.

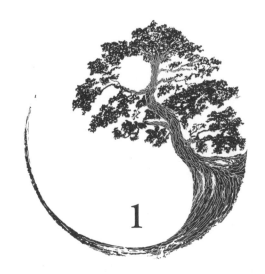

My Unexpected Miracle

As unlikely as it may sound, I was making plans to write a book and make a documentary film about my patients' healing miracles when I found myself suddenly thrust into a series of unexpected, life-changing events that resulted in my own desperate need for a miracle. This is my personal journey from factors that led to my own health crisis, to my complete brokenness, to my awareness and wholeness of a total transformation. This is something I never expected to write about, but I am because I feel it is important to share. Obscure life factors can affect any of us at any time, and they can be destructive on many levels. My journey might help you understand how each element of superconscious healing nurtures the others and how the wholeness, the completeness, of body, mind, and soul, merged with the superconsciousness of the Universe, can make miracles real.

While I don't think I ever took it for granted, I did grow pretty accustomed to a good life that was highlighted by exceptional health. I was rather proud of the fact that I hadn't needed or taken any pharmaceutical or over-the-counter drug for over fifty years. I ate extremely well, took nutritional supplements, and exercised regularly. Then, in the early spring of 2014, virtually out of the blue, things took a swift and decided turn. I began to experience a variety of disturbing symptoms. I noticed that my mobility, especially on my left side, was becoming marginally restricted. I walked three miles a day, four days a week, so I was extremely attuned to my gait and form, and from time to time I could feel my left arm swing with less verve on my morning walks. I began to notice that by the time the end of the workweek rolled around, I felt markedly drained both physically and mentally. The conditions were slowly worsening, and a host of other symptoms gradually began to appear.

By the winter of 2015, all my joints and muscles had become painfully inflamed. I'd lost eighteen pounds in the span of about three months, even though my diet and calorie intake had remained consistent. My entire nervous system began to feel hypersensitive and agitated. I was anxious and, at times, uncharacteristically panicky. These symptoms persisted and worsened over the next year and a half, and then all at once, in the early summer of 2016, I started to develop hand tremors and was beginning to experience a noticeable diminishment of my motor skills. My once-razor-sharp brain began to struggle with the simplest cognitive challenges. I was having some trouble forming words and speaking with the confidence and fluidity that I'd grown so accustomed to. Suddenly, once-simple tasks like standing erectly, walking, talking, getting dressed (buttoning buttons, tying shoes, and threading a belt), showering, turning over in bed, and cooking meals had become massive challenges. Even though my diet and exercise protocols were optimal, my body was overproducing a flood of highly inflammatory stress hormones that were beating me up. I remember feeling as though my body and mind were betraying me. In fact, this was so much so that by the fall of 2016, I felt as though I no longer knew who I was. The utter sense of dislocation from a core self, once strong and reliable, led to a morose dimming of my spirit.

It was becoming clear to me that I'd become a victim of my own choices. There may well have been biochemical factors contributing to my systemic breakdown, but I couldn't deny that stress, overwork, and self-betrayal were playing a significant role in all this. Amid all these physical and mental challenges, I also had to admit that radical changes in my personal and business lives had catapulted my mental stress to a level ten. I'd recently signed a major publishing deal and managed to push through a tight window of back-to-back book deadlines that amazingly resulted in two best sellers and a Nautilus Book Award for the most visionary book of the year. Both books were swiftly written, produced, and on the shelves within a nine-month period. During that time, I appeared on *The Dr. Oz Show*, as well as a variety of other network television programs, and did hundreds of radio interviews. I was also barnstorming around the country, performing seminars and doing secondary-market interviews while the energy of vajra honed in on me.

There's a unique process of ascension and attainment through purification that, in the esoteric doctrine of Buddha, is called *vajra*, or "the great thunderbolt." It represents a sudden, dramatic shift of energy with the power to lift us up and out of, and to hurl us beyond, our long-suffering karmic evolution. Vajra is like a sudden unexpected shockwave that forever alters the course of our life, as opposed to the gradual process of Sanchita Karma, which prompts us to reach attainment step by step. Vajra propels us, abruptly and without warning, into attainment. The great intensity and shock of vajra can be extremely taxing on the physical body and is, in some cases, life-threatening. In fact, by imposing such a forceful karmic shift, vajra not only creates miracles but can leave us needing one. I was quickly falling into that category.

It was all shaping up to be nothing short of a cataclysmic period in my life. I always subscribed to the philosophy that everything is always on the table, but there was simply no more room on my table. Cause and effect seemed to be out of sequence and spiraling out of control. It was as though every negative effect was giving birth to a new cause that only produced the next set of effects. Many of the karmic decisions that I'd made leading up to that time had amassed to create a tipping point that had now come home to roost. It was obvious to me that I was experiencing a complete reordering of my life. It was as though I was on an installment plan, paying for the karmic debt accumulated from this and all my previous lives.

At home I had a thriving practice. I was seeing a dozen patients a day, did a weekly radio show and a bimonthly nutrition segment on Boston's Fox television affiliate. All of these strange physical changes were a backdrop to a very demanding life, and I simply didn't have time for them. Worse, my personal life was hitting a most unforgiving wall.

One realization I had of significant importance had to do with self-betrayal. Regrettably, I'd compromised many of my most integral needs throughout much of my life. I'd become programmed to give, but I did not know how to receive. Growing up the last of four in a family environment where harmony was a precious and rare commodity, I was accustomed to taking on the role of the peacemaker, even as a young child. And though I was born to heal, growing up having to be a healer took a lot out of me. My needs often took a back seat to a host of ongoing dramas. Subsequently, many of the relationships I'd formed throughout my life were unconscious reactions from my wounded-child self, rather than the conscious action of my higher self. I'd become selfless to the point of debilitation. I was the initiator, the enabler, the caregiver, and the apologizer. Now I had to contend with the cumulative karma from years of genuine self-denial. I felt that I was genuinely a good person because I diligently tried to be good to everyone. Everyone, that is, but myself. I was beginning to realize that in order to become a great man, I would have to learn to be honest, appreciative, and good to myself.

I was learning the hard way that the selfless suffer unto themselves. When I was in free fall, many of those I'd chosen to surround myself with were either not willing or not capable of rendering unconditional support. Moreover, there were even those, some who were closest to me, who actually chose to pile on when I was down. Words like *friend* and *lover* lost their clarification during that time. I learned that until you truly love and befriend yourself, you simply can't trust your own judgment to create healthy relationships. I knew that this was about me, and the plain truth was that my spirit had been dis-eased for so long that my body was now riddled with disease.

Regardless, something needed to change, and I decided to take immediate action. I felt that this was likely a case of something fairly elusive like Lyme disease and/or a retrovirus, and because, in my view, the world of orthodox medicine struggles with such nebulous conditions, I decided to initiate my healing process by working on myself. I began comprehensively assessing myself through my own system of energy diagnosis. According to my analysis, the causal root of my symptoms was an acute neurological inflammation from a chronic bacterial infection, coupled with accompanying retrovirus (chronic RNA viruses that replicates by inserting a DNA copy) and fungal infections from mold exposure. I wondered how this could have come on so swiftly and with such intensity. It was clear that long-term stress and self-betrayal had all but obliterated my immune resistance. I remember thinking that it was imperative that I manage this dire situation, as my condition was worsening with each passing day.

I immediately began following a strict anti-inflammatory diet. My dietary adherence went from 85 to 100 percent compliance. I made sure that absolutely no form of dairy, wheat, yolks, corn, nuts, seeds, fermented food, alcohol, or processed sugar came within a scintilla of my palate. I began supplementing with 1,100 parts per million of antibacterial colloidal silver, 3,600 milligrams of Monolaurin to fight the retrovirus, and homeopathic yeast-mold drops for the mold (fungal) exposure. Despite these initial efforts, my condition continued to decline. On top of the disease, I was dealing with both die-off and Herxheimer effects, which meant that as I killed off the infectious microbes, they were releasing toxins that were dumping directly into my bloodstream. I was beginning to get the idea that this was no ordinary health crisis, and I felt like I was up against mutated, stealth microbes.

I gave in and contacted a medical doctor friend because instinctively I realized this was a case where allopathic, traditional Western medicine and naturopathic medicine can complement each other. My plan was to have my blood thoroughly screened by a reliable laboratory. My doctor performed a comprehensive series of blood screenings. The results revealed that I did indeed test positive for Lyme disease (neuroborreliosis), myco-plasma infection, which is a bacterial infection, and Epstein-Barr virus, which is a stress-induced virus. I frequently enjoy hiking in the woods and apparently managed to get a tick bite during one of my excursions. With all the stress in my hectic life and the immunodeficiency issue caused by the bacterial and viral infections, I was especially susceptible to the effects of that small creature's bite.

I left no stone unturned regarding forms of treatment. Between 2015 and 2018, I cycled through fifty to sixty natural and pharmaceutical medi-cines and employed the services of medical doctors, nurse practitioners, laser therapists, acupuncturists, chiropractors, massage therapists, Chi Gong practitioners, Reiki therapists, psychologists, energy healers, and psychics. I was desperate. Despite the various therapies I employed, the unceasing physical, mental, and emotional pain that I was enduring only intensified.

By 2017 the pain had dramatically increased, and I began to lose strength, mobility, and balance in both my upper and lower body. By the autumn of 2017, I could barely walk. I didn't have enough strength in my back and legs to even hold myself up. I felt as though my muscles were dying.

Due only to the power of my spirit and commitment to my patients, I managed to make it to work every day and somehow found a way to function, though barely, during this period. Patients would come in, and I would counsel them as best I could from a seated position and in great pain. It was more difficult than I can ever adequately explain. I chose to be completely honest with my patients about what I was going through. Every moment of every workday, I had to fight through the intense misery, pain, and yes, even shame. I am a deeply spiritual man but still so very mortal. I had yet to fully overcome my human pride. I worked very hard to get to where I was in my life, and I was still attached to the trappings of material success, physical beauty, and ego-based empowerment. It was clear to me that this was a time in my life when the Universe expected me to overcome those egocentric limitations.

With rapidly diminishing strength, balance, and mobility, not to mention depression, anxiety, and panic, I felt forced to socially cut myself off from the world. Out of necessity, I began to withdraw deeper into my inner sanctum. I recall flashing back to earlier times when I abhorred being alone. This time being alone turned out to be a very transformative time because I had an opportunity to review my soul and spirit evolution. I came to realize that by allowing my lofty goals and visions to overwork me and turn me into a "human doing" rather than a human being, I'd betrayed myself, and in the understanding of that, I was able to forgive myself. Through meditation and prayer, I managed to finally develop a deep and loving relationship with my once-forgotten self. This was clearly an equalizing time of my life when I was expected to learn to love being alone with myself, a time when I could exorcise any and all my demons of self-contempt. I could actually feel that as my body was contracting, my soul and spirit were expanding.

I'd always resonated with the Hindu belief that everything comes down to karma and moksha. Everything we think, say, and do results either as karma (negative consequences of our actions) or as moksha (liberation from suffering). I realized that at that point in my life, many of my karmically ill-fated decisions were returning to haunt me. My unconscious mind was hiding deep inner turbulence that reverberated through my soul. I realized that my dialogue with self was obscured by the influence of the deep wounds from my earlier life. My dysfunctional relationship with myself had resulted in unhealthy relationships with others. My spirit was dis-eased, and my body could no longer hold up under the strain. I was on an installment plan paying dearly for my moksha.

On the evening of July 2, 2018, my partner, Fabiola, was my dinner guest. We enjoyed each other's company for several hours and began to wrap up our time together at approximately eleven o'clock.

She left my apartment, and as was my custom, I didn't deadbolt my front door until after I returned from getting myself ready for bed. Immediately after she left, I stepped into the bathroom, and as I did, my balance became very unsteady. The next thing I knew I was face down on the cold, hard tile of the bathroom floor. Worst of all, I couldn't move a muscle. As I lay there motionless, I was forced to both breathe in and swallow a mix of toxic bathroom cleaning agents that I knocked over when I fell. I literally could not move my head out of the way. I was trapped in my own body. I remember thinking, *Am I paralyzed? Do I have a concussion? Am I bleeding? What just happened to me?*

Whenever Fabiola and I visit with each other, we always text each other with a good night wish before retiring. I wasn't able to reach my phone because I couldn't move. As I lay helpless on the floor, I hoped and prayed that both the absence of a final good night text and an unlocked front door would result in my discovery. I remembered that just prior to Fabiola's departure, she and I had engaged in a three-hour conversation about "needless worry." I couldn't help but wonder if the nature of that conversation might negatively influence my chances for a swift rescue. As the hours passed, I slowly began to realize that this dilemma had a divinely purposeful nature to it.

I had endured nearly five years of chronic, excruciating pain, inflammation, and overwhelming fatigue, as well as profound mental and emotional debilitation. Now, I found myself completely benumbed on a bathroom floor, inhaling toxic chemicals. I was vacillating between wondering if I was going to die that night and not knowing if I wanted to live anymore anyway. I was paralyzed, and the thought of living in a mind without a body was devastating to me.

As I lay there despondent, I was tormented by the very deepest and darkest of thoughts. I remember thinking at that time that I had a crucial question to answer, and that was, How is my spirit? I came to realize that my spirit was all I had during those years of hell, and now, under these acutely dire circumstances, I needed to know if it was still determined or even willing to live. At that point, I truly didn't know the answer. As my physical body lay broken and trapped on a bathroom floor, my entire inner being struggled with that question. Every second was an eternity. This was the lowest point in my life, and it felt as if all the light had been extinguished.

Do I want to live? I asked myself.

I honestly don't know was the answer.

There was even one point when I felt ready, willing, and able to give up my life and liberate my spirit from my body.

Then, inexplicably, I felt my spirit suddenly rise up above my body. In what seemed like an instant, I saw my entire life pass before me. At first, I was convinced that I was indeed dying and that my spirit was, in fact, leaving my body. Then, all at once, as if my voice belonged to someone else, I started screaming at the top of my lungs. "Help! Can anybody hear me?"

By asking for help, I got my answer! My spirit wanted to live!

Nobody heard me, but it didn't matter. I'd fallen into a bottomless black hole, but now I knew I'd begun my ascent. As I lay there motionless on that hard tile floor, I had made the most important decision I'd ever made in my entire life, and I made it with an unparalleled degree of certitude. I felt a cataclysmic shift within me, from desperation to determination. I decided that I was going to go ahead with the writing of this book and producing *The Way of Miracles* film, and if need be, I would write, conduct interviews, present lectures and seminars, go on book tours, and take patient appointments from a wheelchair. I was suddenly steadfast and resolute about living an uncompromised life! I felt a desire to live as never before. Moreover, my spirit understood that I had to fall in order to rise and that declination and ascension are inseparable.

It had finally become clear to me that I had to reach this low point in my life as part of my transformational destiny. I knew that I would have to confront many difficult circumstances and people in my life. Lying on that floor, I suddenly understood just how precious my entire life was and how much I needed me! Vajra, the great thunderbolt, had come to awaken me to me! There were still more questions than answers, but the most important question had been answered by my spirit. I wanted to live with a determination to be fully alive, regardless of whether or not my body was capable.

Finally, after a fourteen-and-a-half-hour eternity, I heard Fabiola's voice calling to me. As it turned out, she did indeed feel unsettled about my having never sent that good night text and was suspicious that something was wrong. As I heard her voice, I breathed a sigh of relief, and I remember thinking, *Thank God I didn't deadbolt the front door!*

I called back to her, and she entered the bathroom. The first thing I heard her say was that there was no sign of bleeding. She then attempted to gently lift me up but couldn't. I was absolute dead weight. I asked her to call my son, Nick, who was at work at the time. He arrived in approximately forty-five minutes, gently lifted my immobile body, and carried me to the bed. I spent the next ten days in convalescence at home. This was no small task as I was completely unable to move my body. I thank God for those dearest to me. Fabiola, Nick, my daughter, Vanessa, and my friends Siobhan, Jim, Lisa, and Kelly led the way for the next ten days. I had to be carried to the bathroom, shopped for, cooked for, fed, shaved, bathed, and dressed, and when none of them could be there for me, they made sure that someone else was. They took care of all my bodily needs, but more than that, they fed my soul with love and made certain that my spirit remained elevated. It was their care and compassion that brought me through to the other side of my darkest hour.

As that first week passed, everyone, including me, had serious doubts as to whether I would ever fully recover. I was paralyzed and wondered if this was going to be a permanent state. During many deeply personal moments, of which there were many, I prayed and meditated to cultivate superconsciousness. I was determined to program my being for a miracle healing.

At the ten-day mark, I was still immobile and had only experienced slight improvement. Due to my holistic background, I'm not inclined to use pharmaceutical medicine, nor am I inclined to go to hospitals; moreover, I didn't believe that there was a soul on earth who could talk me into such a prospect. I know that sounds crazy to some, but that is who I am. Nonetheless, following some intensely sobering conversations with Fabiola, I deferred to a plan to get my partially paralyzed body out of bed, down three flights of stairs, into a car, and off to the nearest hospital. I knew that tall task was going to require a miracle. Nick had to carry me, and each and every step down the three flights of stairs of my apartment building was a journey unto itself. It's a truly humbling experience to have your brain generating all the energy it can muster, messaging your legs to move . . . and absolutely no electrical connection. Somehow, we got it done, and soon I was comfortably settled in a wheelchair, checking into the hospital.

The hospital personnel ran a comprehensive series of blood tests and brain scans. My vitals were continually being monitored, even to the aggravating point of interfering with my sleep and rest. I remember the shock of hearing that I weighed in at 134 pounds! My average weight had always been about 162.

After a day or so, a team of doctors and neurologists was evaluating me. I explained to them all that blood tests previously ordered by my doctor had discovered that I was suffering from a type of Lyme disease, mycoplasma, and Epstein-Barr virus. The hospital doctors simply didn't want to hear anything about any such nouveau diagnostic contentions. Orthodox medicine is simply not prepared to accept the evolving reality of these "New Age" illnesses. They are more drawn to the idea of focusing on symptoms. What classic disease does the patient's symptoms reflect? Then, they simply prescribe pharmaceutical medicine to shut down the expression of the symptoms.

Neuroborreliosis is a type of Lyme disease, and its symptoms mimic Parkinson's disease. Without a spinal tap, and based solely on symptoms, doctors tend to simply diagnose such conditions as Parkinson's. This is exactly what they did with me. They then prescribed Sinemet, a medication that increases the brain's levels of dopamine, an organic chemical that functions as both a hormone and neurotransmitter. It's responsible for the communication between nerve cells in the brain, especially in the substantia nigra, a body movement center.

Among the many blood tests my doctor ran weeks prior was a dopamine test. I found it interesting that the test revealed that I actually had elevated levels of dopamine! This could only mean that I wasn't distributing and absorbing it efficiently. Instead, my body was depositing it in a way that rendered it unavailable for my brain. I knew I wasn't going to get anywhere with the medical orthodoxy on these issues. While I was pleased that the Sinemet seemed to help with my symptoms, I more or less put the diagnosis debate on hold.

After spending five days in the hospital, I was taken by ambulance to a rehabilitation clinic, where I spent a week learning how to walk again. My doctors at the hospital were certain that I'd need a minimum of two full weeks of rehab, plus ongoing physical therapy on a bi- or triweekly basis once I returned home. I was told that I would likely not be able to work again. My vision was also very different. But I had communicated with my soul, and I knew what I wanted. I was determined to walk again, go home in one week, rehab at home by myself, and get back to work in three weeks.

I checked into rehab late on a Friday afternoon. A small part of me was a little depressed as I thought back to the many enjoyable Friday evenings and weekends I'd spent in my life. This overwhelming chapter in my life was unlike anything I'd ever experienced. That didn't matter because the biggest part of me remained all business! I was determined to walk again and soon! I couldn't wait to hit the classes in the rehab gym. In fact, I barely got started when I doubled up on my rehab schedule. I was present and accounted for in every class I signed up for. While clearly impressed with my effort, the instructors were doing their best to temper my expectations. In fact, every healthcare professional I worked with during those two weeks had a vision very unlike mine. I was headed in a very different direction because I was coming from a very different place.

At first, I commuted back and forth from class and up and down the halls in a wheelchair. Just prior to my first class, I was assigned a walker for my exercises. I found this depressing but remained determined to accomplish my goals. I must admit, those first classes were demanding and exhausting. It took every ounce of strength in me to walk fifteen to twenty feet with a walker, and it took all of the balance I could muster to do it in a straight line. I remember feeling envious, and bit resentful, as I watched the instructors demonstrating the exercises with ease. As I watched them, I thought, *I absolutely refuse to go on this way! I will go on to experience a complete recovery!*

During my second day at rehab, I began to reflect on the miracle recoveries that so many of my severely and terminally ill patients had experienced over the past three and a half decades. While there were secondary reasons for the miraculous turnaround of each of them, there was always one pivotal common denominator: the spirit of superconsciousness permeated our healing work together. When you get right down to it, that's the key source of miracle-making magic. *Now it was time for my miracle*, I thought.

I engaged in superconscious prayer, meditation, and trance later that evening. The next day I made my greatest progress in physical therapy. My mobility and balance had taken a quantum leap forward overnight! As the week went on, I continued my superconscious cultivation, and my progress continued at an astonishing rate. I was well on my way to creating my miracle. About three weeks later, I was at last able to walk a bit. At that time, I added some powerful, antimicrobial herbal medicines, namely, banderol, cumanda, burbur, houttuynia, and oregano oil.

After strictly following this regime for eighteen months, I was completely recovered. While I do still experience some occasional minor symptoms, I've progressed from acute pain and paralysis to once again being fully functional. I now walk eight miles per week at a pretty moderate clip, and while there are many important factors that went into my miraculous turnaround, I attribute my success to my day-to-day dedication to superconscious prayer, meditation, and trance manifest.

Soul Reminders I Needed to Experience

Like so many others, I perceived the events of my life as separate and without an intertwined connection. Prior to my unexpected healing miracle, I lived my life unaware of any real connection between brokenness and wholeness. I only recognized the pain that resulted from my lack of connection to self. I didn't understand that being broken created an opportunity to receive and be filled.

But, true to the Universe's law of wholeness, the gaping wounds of my brokenness created openness that made room for my transformational growth and liberation. I finally realized that the more broken I was, the more opened up I became. The greater the degree and depth of my distress, the greater my need was to be filled full. In the end, it was my agonizing brokenness that gave birth to my deepest fulfillment.

Discovering the Wholeness of Everything

Many sacred doctrines attempt to drive home the point that suffering is not without purpose. I had heard the message a thousand times, but it was only through a superconsciousness miracle moment that I came to truly understand suffering as an inseparable part of a greater whole, which includes healing and rebirth.

Conversations about brokenness bring to mind suffering. But from the superconscious perspective, there's a sacred quality to brokenness. In order for us to appreciate such a quality, we must first come to understand that breaking is not an ending but a continuation. Life is like a river that flows ever forward. In every moment of each lifetime, we give birth to a new, ever-unfolding "self." As we grow, we break through and extend beyond a comfortable, womblike threshold of familiarity. Moving out of comfort to the unknown tends to be destabilizing because with it there is always some type of breakage.

Due to its ego-stripping nature, brokenness brings about purification. It eradicates all semblance of willpower and leaves room only for the true self. With the ego removed from the equation, all that remains is our soul, spirit, and heart. Although it might feel like an ending, brokenness isn't. In fact, it represents a karmic continuum that begins and cycles over, and over, and over again with new beginnings.

Nothing avails the truth quite like brokenness. It absolves us of all grand illusions, leaving only a naked veracity that cuts to the bone. The darkness that appears to accompany brokenness is but a mirage that gives way to the resplendent light. Absolute brokenness brings you to a place where you are one with truth.

I mistook my brokenness as the beginning of an ending. It took me some time to know that there are no endings and nothing ever dies; everything merely changes. I had to find a way to make sense of all the changes that were destined to follow my brokenness. My miracle helped me make sense of these changes. I discovered that brokenness doesn't take away anything. Instead, it gives. It gives the ultimate gift of awakening us to the presence of our true soul nature. Through the cracks of what may appear as absolute destruction shines the eternal light that reflects the self, which we truly are.

I have worked with many patients once terminally ill, now successfully healed, who got down on their knees and thanked their past illness for teaching them who they truly were. They chose to treat their illness as a sacred gift. They understood that breaking is an action; brokenness is a state, a state that we arrive at after extensive breaking. Nobody breaks once—we break constantly—but only so that we might constantly be made new.

The flow of life is not linear; it's circular. Therefore, every state of brokenness will ultimately evolve to a state of wholeness. It was my tendency to perceive unfolding events in my life as a series of isolated, disconnected freeze-frames. I believed that whatever was to happen would just happen unto itself, without any sequential connection to what happened before it.

My miracle experience inspired me to become more aligned with superconsciousness, and superconsciousness opened me up to the integral interconnectedness of all events in my life, eternally. I now have a greater appreciation for the cyclical genesis of all and everything. I understand that brokenness ultimately transmutes to a state of unbrokenness by way of oneness. There is ultimately no line of separation between the two. There is only wholeness.

Acknowledging the Cycles of Life

And so it was, on a cold bathroom floor, I suddenly found myself engaged in a profoundly compelling conversation with death itself. In that moment, I awkwardly attempted to dispel any part of the great mystery that I could and was prompted to ask all the standard questions: What would my death be like? Would it be painful? Would I feel lost after I crossed into the unknown? Would I still be some semblance of me, at least in my mind? Of course, these questions all represented my response to death from the personal consciousness perspective. But I discovered that I also had an option to respond to the prospect of my death from a more superconsciousness vantage point.

Dying is a process that is initiated at birth and reaches a crescendo with the cessation of our mortality. There is no beginning to its endlessness. There is no terminus to the absolute absence of its presence. For all our intellectual sophistication and from a personal consciousness perspective, we know very little about death, for with death comes an unfailing amnesia. All we think we know about death is only what we've been able to glean from life and living. Beyond that, it's a veritable free-for-all. Your guess is as good as mine. Most, but not all, view it with negativity.

Like brokenness, death, in all its formless manifestations, is perfectly aligned with life. Yes, even death is part of a greater wholeness. When I say "all its formless manifestations," I'm referring to the fact that long before we actually pass on physically, we die a thousand deaths mentally, emotionally, and spiritually. While those thousand nonphysical deaths may have resulted in profound brokenness, what have we learned from them? Do you feel as though you've come to really understand the lessons of these agonizing states?

Have you ever felt imprisoned in such a deeply darkened moment that you suddenly found yourself engaged in an intimate conversation with the spirit of death? I did, and in so doing, I learned that there was no greater way for me to fully come alive than to entertain a conversation with death about the way I was living my life.

Spiritually, *death* is a word that speaks to transmutation. Materially, it suggests a baseless void that reaches far beyond brokenness. The great force of the event that it represents lies in its forcefulness. It thrusts each and every one of us into the ultimate transformation, the details of which remain a mystery even though I'd recently found myself completely conversant with it.

Several years ago I had an interesting conversation with a practicing Christian about a friend of hers who'd just passed away. I offered her my condolences, whereupon she remarked, "Oh, there's nothing sad about his passing. He was a devout Christian, and he was a believer who'd accepted Christ as his savior. His funeral and wake will be something of a victory celebration for his saved soul."

This made a strong impression on me. The profound truth of the association between death and victory was an awakening. This positive perspective of death that is shared by many world religions and spiritual disciplines is radically different than the standard material Western view.

Here in the West, the very essence of life is rooted in materialism. As a material culture, we are form based. If there's no physical body, there's no baseline for life as we know it, and if there's no baseline for life, the result can only be no-thing-ness. Although Westerners may talk about soul and the prospect of its journey through eternity, we struggle to get beyond the conversation. In much of the modern West, death is simply seen as the end of life, a proposition for which there is no cause for celebration. In the materialistic world, celebrations are dedicated exclusively to life and are mostly reflective of productivity, growth, and success.

The personal consciousness of the Western mind is inclined to separate beginnings from endings. Living is synonymous with success, and death is tantamount to failure. In the East, there is no difference between life and death. They believe they are representative of one whole continuum, where life naturally flows into death and death gives birth to new life. These diametrically opposite perspectives reveal stark contrasts in consciousness. Personal consciousness is inclined to adopt the corporeal viewpoint. Superconsciousness, however, reflects the wisdom to understand beginnings and endings as a whole-istic perpetuity of opposites endlessly pouring themselves into each other.

With superconsciousness, all that lives evolves from a state of something to a state of nothing, which initiates the infinite field of everything. Every particle of life is simultaneously a reflection of something, nothing, and everything. Superconsciousness sees right through illusions. It understands that, just as birth is the ultimate illusion about beginnings, death is the ultimate illusion about the appearance of endings.

Personal consciousness makes us believers in endings and losses. When someone we know and love dies, we often speak of "losing" them. Superconsciousness knows that in death nothing is ever lost. It understands that it's about every soul finding its way through eternity.

The personal consciousness view of death, not unlike its view of life, is profoundly self-limiting, if not debilitating. Its depiction of self is very much a stand-alone and independent entity. It sees self as completely absent of any integral connection with the Universe. That concept of self, mired in bleak isolation, powerlessness, and impermanence, is disconnected from the natural dictates of universal order.

The personal consciousness perception of self is based largely on weaknesses, rather than on strengths. It embraces mortality. It believes in the force of our will, rather than the power of soul. It honors achievement rather than attainment. Arguably, the greatest weakness of personal consciousness is its misperception of death, for this misunderstanding of death profoundly weakens the capacity to live life to its fullest.

If we are locked into personal consciousness, we move through our days in denial, as though we're going to have them forever. We resent and defy the natural process of aging because it represents gradual death. We attach and cling to virtually every material aspect of life, hanging on as though once this incarnation ends, everything will forever fade to black.

We belong to a techno-mechanistic tribe. We are a cultural experiment defined by our collective vision of success. Never before has a society been so consumed by its drive for material advancement. We've all been weaned on a philosophy espousing the highest level of socioeconomic growth and monetary advancement. From our earliest beginnings, our process is a progressive one, as we advance from one year's achievement baseline to the next. Once our schooling is over, this progressive evolvement continues with our work. As we increasingly expand our knowledge and expertise at work, we attain greater status, for which we are rewarded. Our life is all about growth, progression, and reward, until we die.

Through all those years of cultivating a living and achieving success, there's always been a shadow of darkness lurking in the backdrop of our life. Not unlike the six-hundred-pound gorilla in the corner of the room, it's virtually impossible to ignore. Nothing sabotages success and life quite like death. While we might choose to ignore it, we remain powerless in the bold face of its truth. There's simply not enough addictive distraction available for us to deny its presence. It's a stark reality we simply must surrender to in order for us to move through the evolution of a more real success.

To embrace the totality of wholeness, we should expand the consciousness with which we attempt to understand death. Through meditation, prayer, and the merger of the subconscious mind with the collective Universal consciousness, we engage our immortal self. By cultivating superconsciousness, we transform into that self that transcends death. It is superconsciousness that energetically transports our being to the immortal state where the mere actualization of our eternal nature exposes the great myth of death.

We are as morning drops of dew, once clinging to the velvety petals of a rose, then evaporated by the heat of the noonday sun, and forever destined to return with the rising mists of the midnight moon.

We fall to rise again, just as we return to awaken . . .

As mortals, we age and die. As immortals, we evolve and ascend. We only die to live, and we only fall to rise. We come into this temporal existence destined to fall hard and often because it's only by falling hard and often that we're driven to the spiritual ascension that leads to the highest attainment. Our greatest measure is not determined by our material achievement but rather by our spiritual attainment. Ascension and attainment are the natural results of the cause and effect of a protracted karmic evolution, but for a precious few, they're about being thrust into the torrent of a transformational shift. Such was the case regarding my miracle story.

Understanding the Wholeness of Everything

In accordance with most ancient spiritual traditions, attainment is defined as the cultivation of consciousness aligned with the creator. Moreover, it's generally accepted by most traditions that our principal reason for living is only so that we can evolve, transform, and ultimately reach the highest level of spiritual attainment. Attainment is the ultimate destiny of every soul, most commonly accessed through the step-by-step ascension of spirit through what the Hindus call Sanchita Karma, or gradual purification from the cleansing of mortal cause and effect. While Sanchita Karma brings us closer to attainment, it is an unending process. By continually facing and working though the many challenges of karma during our many lifetimes, we ultimately evolve in consciousness and ascend in spirit, on our way to reaching attainment.

A natural gravity-like response governs our karmic relationship with pain and suffering. The more intense our pain and suffering are, the greater our need is to ascend and attain. If we choose to resist and deny, the forces of our pain and suffering will continue to mass until they are responded to naturally. This is like a great universal fail-safe that guarantees a spiritual evolution, tempered by process. Our pain masses and deepens, and mortal solutions fail again and again, as a sacred gravity positions us more in the direction of a deeper spiritual cleansing. The greater our karmic repression, the more inevitable the likelihood we'll be forced to contend with the great thunderbolt.

It's important to remember that vajra isn't a phenomenon that randomly appears in our lives. We unconsciously create it. *Unconsciously* is the keyword here. It is the intense pain and suffering that accompany our karma that generate the power that energizes the great thunderbolt.

Many are deeply perplexed as to the specific nature of the karmic conflicts they've come to contend with in this life. We awaken to each morning and engage in the rituals of each new day. We may not be aware of the details regarding the unfolding of our deeper karmic process, but we're all too aware of the pain and suffering that accompany it. By attempting to deaden ourselves to the torment, we only serve to intensify it. As one day gives way to the next, pain and suffering masses on the unconscious level. The internal pressure within builds and builds, until all at once, it generates a powerful cleansing force, and it can open up a whole new vista and create a pathway to what is perhaps the greatest of all miracles: superconscious transformation.

While it's certainly true that the prayer, meditation, and trance manifest that I practiced during the darkest period of my soul were important vehicles for manifesting my superconscious healing miracle, *the most* important way to cultivate superconsciousness is to live in the constant state of mindfulness.

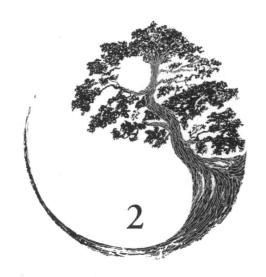

2

Consciousness

What makes a miracle? The answer is simple. You do!

Miracles happen around us all the time. Some are small and common while others are grand and exceptional. Still, most of us don't know how to define them, recognize them, or manifest them because most of us don't believe in them.

I used to be one who fit perfectly into that category.

I grew up in a conservative, middle-class American neighborhood in an unconscious culture. I was lost if a discussion deviated from mainstream thought. Like most everyone else, I believed that if a topic couldn't pass a five-sensory, three-dimensional thump on it—that is, a logic test—it wasn't worth examining. Extrapolation of a theory or a creative spark that was nothing more than a concept was a complete waste of time. Or so I thought.

But my life took a radical turn. I shared an interest in natural medicine and nutrition with my father, and by my late twenties, I was a graduate student working on a master's degree in nutrition and a doctorate in health.

I finished school and began working as a holistic practitioner. My medicine of choice was food, specifically, applied nutritional therapy. I set up a modest practice in the back of a hair salon in the quaint New England village of Cohasset, Massachusetts. Almost immediately, remarkable things began to happen to my patients and to me. I began to pay attention to these simple miracles that were transpiring on many levels. As small demonstrations of miracles grew and became more numerous, I slowly began to see things differently until my awareness encompassed a new reality. Inconceivable occurrences unfolded as miracles grew from a tiny trickle to a steady stream until I could no longer ignore them. I had to know how they came into reality for the people I work with and for myself.

Awareness

Are you aware that you *are* pure awareness? Everything that you and I exist within informs and expands our consciousness. Our interactions with people, nature, inanimate objects, everything that informs our five senses and our knowledge base defines our awareness and, therefore, our consciousness. But in order for our consciousness to be our reality, it must be observed either objectively or subjectively. It requires a witness. Through our awareness of and by our observations of all of these interactions, we make a conscious determination that defines what we believe to be reality. Consciousness, then, becomes the most important aspect of life as it defines what we think is truly real.

What happens if reality is not determined by observation? What if the witness isn't aware? If we are basically unconscious of our consciousness, reality lacks sentience because it holds no essence or energy.

Consciousness and awareness are inseparable. While the Universe is created from consciousness, awareness is the faculty through which it perceives itself. There can be no consciousness without observed awareness.

But being aware of our consciousness opens a world of possibilities that range from the mundane to the transcendental. Unfortunately, the majority of the population remains unconscious of extreme thoughts and rarely examines the myriad questions that can be posed to help us expand our awareness.

Theoretical queries are a spark of creativity that broadens perception beyond routine thought. Have you ever wondered about abstract concepts such as:

- Is the universe consciousness?

- Is it aware of its consciousness?

- What about trees, rocks, blades of grass, and droplets of dew? Do they have consciousness?

Questions like those obviously blossom into mind-boggling theories while answers to them become less defined and more speculative. But does that mean that they should not be explored? We exist in a culture that rarely places importance on matters that we can't thump on, yet these esoteric contemplations can expand our awareness and, in turn, our consciousness. And that broadens the reality in which we exist.

However, it's important to begin with a raw concept. In the most bare, basic sense, I prefer to simply think of consciousness as the energy generated by awareness.

It reveals and infuses everything with *being-ness*, which is the quality of being in existence. The observation of *is-ness* represents the most powerful way we can witness and validate the presence of consciousness.

An example of this might be the first time I looked into the eyes of my newborn children. As they peered back at me, I witnessed the absolute personification of being-ness.

By gazing into my children's eyes during their first moments of life, I awakened to the knowledge that consciousness can't be attained or lost, for it isn't something we possess. It's the sum total of what we are. It is the formless embodiment of our timeless essence. It's the eternity prior to our birth and the perpetuity after our death. Pure consciousness is all we have been and all we will ever be. It's the omnipresence of awareness of all that is.

The human mind is capable of categorizing and producing distinctly different states of consciousness. Each separate state generates its own unique properties, which result in a variety of different capabilities and powers. Each requires awareness of and recognition of their specific qualities to reach the all-encompassing state of superconsciousness, for that represents the alliance of our personal mind with the universal mind. I believe each of us can access and attain this ultimate power through a conversion from personal consciousness to superconsciousness.

By elevating our level of awareness to the degree that we can access and blend with the collective cosmic mind, we naturally inherit a transcendent power that is unlimited. Even though we are all capable of producing random miracles, we also have the ability to consistently produce intentional miracles, which are accomplished by expanding our reality to include the vastness of superconsciousness.

From the perspectives of science, psychology, and the anatomy of the human mind, the four states of awareness representing varied manifestations of consciousness are:

1. The Conscious Mind: Our day-to-day personal awareness

2. The Subconscious Mind: Our stored, forgotten personal awareness, which resides below the conscious level that *can* be recalled

3. The Unconscious Mind: Our stored, repressed personal awareness that resides below the conscious level that *cannot* be recalled

4. The Superconscious Mind: The merger of our consciousness with an infinite, miracle-making universal awareness

The Conscious Mind

The conscious mind represents awareness of, in, and about the present. It includes thoughts, perceptions, sensations, feelings, fantasies, and memories. The conscious mind is often associated with what is subjectively perceived or experienced by a person, called qualia. The brain can form and reorganize synaptic connections. It is capable of processing up to two thousand bits of information per second, providing us with the astonishing capacity to be consciously aware.

Random miracles occur when we exist within the framework of the conscious mind. When something unexplained but amazing happens to us, we don't understand the totality of the energy involved. Instead of being aware of the power within the miracle, we adorn it with a creative adjective and set it aside as a remarkable coincidence.

The Subconscious Mind

The subconscious mind is a part of the mind that does not engage in focused awareness. It is an infinite reservoir of forgotten or stored memories that can, in some instances, be recalled. The subconscious mind doesn't think or reason unto itself; rather, it follows the direction of the conscious mind.

On the upside, it is an extremely fertile part of the mind that can assist with the reprogramming of habits and behaviors. While the conscious mind can process two thousand bits of information per second, the subconscious mind can process and retain 400 billion.

The Unconscious Mind

The unconscious mind is a reservoir of stored past events. But unlike the subconscious, which simply forgets the past, the unconscious mind intentionally blocks the knowledge of the past. Unconscious recall is often difficult, as the mind and body impose a powerful gridlock of self-protection from memories of pain and suffering.

The Superconscious Mind

While their potential and power are without question, the conscious, subconscious, and unconscious minds can in no way be compared to the omniscient superconscious mind.

The superconscious mind represents the blending of our mind with the Universal mind. The result is consciousness that is limitless and boundless. Some think of it as the divine mind. The British poet Alfred, Lord Tennyson was speaking of superconsciousness when he wrote about the state of transcendental wonder.

It is only by propagating this transcendent state of Universal consciousness that we become empowered to generate fields of infinite possibility.

We *can* reach beyond what we think is in our limited grasp. We can reach those immeasurable opportunities by cultivating consciousness that fuses with the Universal mind to attain superconsciousness. That empowerment enables us to radically advance our proficiency to heal and transform.

The first three aspects of consciousness represent action, or "doing" states. Superconsciousness, however, is the one and only state of mind where our will surrenders to the Universal way of things. By disengaging from our limited, finite knowledge, we are able to plug in to the infinite wisdom of the Universe. There the burdensome limitations imposed by human will are nowhere to be found.

There are two primordial energies of the Universe. They are creation and destruction. These are not only recognized in the physical world in which we live but are valid in all energetic forms. This means that every action that is engaged is one or the other, creative or destructive. That includes thought. In fact, every thought ultimately produces a creational power or a destructive force.

Our greatest creational powers are buried within the deepest recesses of our soul, the source of our being that is inextricably tethered to the collective Universal consciousness. Superconsciousness provides the potential to access that unlimited creational power that each of us possesses.

By cultivating a higher awareness and aligning to that, we can inspire a new world culture or ethos: an ethos of miracles. It is only through this emergence of our soulful superconsciousness that we can discover the way of miracles.

The validity of superconsciousness power has often been observed by science, and growing evidence continues to indicate that the power it wields is, in fact, miraculous.

In 1982, Dr. Herbert Benson headed up a series of studies that examined the effects of superconsciousness. One of the studies, sponsored by Harvard Medical School, set out to observe the superconscious powers of Tibetan monks in the Himalayas as they performed a meditation called Tummo yoga.[1] This powerful meditative exercise is believed to help the monks generate such concentrated power that they are able to manifest an energy capable of drying their freshly washed, soaking wet robes while wearing them in their frigid mountain monastery.

The monks laundered their robes as Benson's crew recorded the indoor temperature of forty-nine degrees Fahrenheit. The monks sat in the full lotus position and began practicing their mind-altering yoga. Within five minutes, the team noted that the camera lenses had fogged up, and the crew had to continually wipe away the condensation. The scientists reported that in a mere thirty minutes from the beginning of the experiment, the monks and their robes were completely warm and dry.

Tibetan monks know that unlimited power is the direct result of the unification of consciousness with the Universal mind. They realize that by cultivating the flow of superconscious energy, they are afforded access to transcendent experiences beyond the normal or physically accepted reality. Through training, they have become masters of creating the perfect emptiness, an open vacuum endlessly being filled full of infinity. Such a flow is a natural byproduct of the superconscious.

The superconscious way of things is principally about the accessibility of unlimited power through universal unification. We're all part of a unified Universe sharing one infinite source of integral energy.

Regardless of our accessibility to such power, there is still an important decision that we each must make. Will we insist on drawing our energy from the finite force of our own willful ego? Or will it come from the infinite wellspring of the infinite Universe?

We *are* the Universe. And we, like the Tibetan monks, can learn to unify the personal mind with the divine Universal mind and remain tapped into its inexhaustible resources. The divine Universal mind is a natural, benevolent power that is abundant and unlimited. It cannot be generated or fabricated by human will. It can only be acquired by reaching the highest state of awareness.

The Transcendent Power of our Being-ness

Imagine an infinite pool of transparent awareness. When all that exists within that infinite pool is reflected to us, we change the field of personal consciousness to the field of Universal consciousness. In this transformed state of being-ness, we have the capacity to access and utilize supreme manifestation because our energy emanates from the soul. The essence of our soul identity represents our extraordinary divine nature.

We are not just ordinary beings; we are extraordinary, and we need to stop labeling and thinking of ourselves in such a limited perspective. Our most intrinsic roots reveal that we are composed of the structures of experience and consciousness. The acronym CHNOPS stands for carbon, hydrogen, nitrogen, oxygen, phosphorus, and sulfur, which together make up the building blocks of life that are found in the human body. According to a news release from Ohio State University's Center for Cosmology and Astroparticle Physics, humans and the galaxy we belong to are made up of the same type of atoms.[2]

Although these elements may be in different proportions, you and I share identical elements with every star in the universe!

We belong to this unified mosaic that's filled with a magical quality and woven together from its microcosmic core to its incalculable macrocosm. Even though each of us is absolutely unique, everything, including each of us, is an undivided part of the other. From the smallest known life form called the nanobe (a bacterium) to a black hole with over four million times the mass of our sun, there is a unifying property that exists in all. This principle common denominator is what I call "the currency of the Universe." That currency is consciousness. Far beyond and deep within our matter, we reflect an animating, interconnecting presence that defines our existence. The term *reflect* is important because we can't have or, for that matter, lose consciousness; we simply are consciousness.

The content of our consciousness defines the quality of our experiences. Qualia, which are defined as subjective conscious experiences, generally capture a snapshot of consciousness in action. Qualia are the perceived personal mental state or distinctive reaction to stimuli that might include pain, smell, taste, or even colors. However, the compelling mystery hiding deep within the concept prompts a more thorough investigation.

This mystery is deeper than those things that generate sensations, emotions, thoughts, dreams, and visions. In this case, the mystery is a non-action state of being that also flows into the boundless stream of consciousness just as qualia does. In that space, we can feel fully present and clear, and we are free to experience the flow of pure awareness. In this domain of heightened realization, we become the witness of our own experiences. It is in this state that we can merge into, and ultimately become one with, our immortal source. The simple act of observation allows this perfect Universal action to manifest. It is the observer, the witness within each of us, that knows the way of miracles.

Miracle Making

The characteristic spirit of a culture, era, or community as manifested in its beliefs, ethics, emotions, and aspirations is referred to as *ethos*. It more or less reflects the baseline of a culture, its philosophy, ideology, and mindset. It also reveals the margins that define the perception of reality and what we generally believe to be possible.

Ethos varies significantly from culture to culture and from person to person. As times change, both cultural and personal attitudes naturally shift and expand or contract. Ethos changes accordingly. Quite often what was once believed to be impossible evolves into possibilities and even probabilities. With the concept of ethos in mind, I pose two questions to you:

1. Do you believe you can access a higher power?

2. If you believe a higher power exists, do you also believe that you can channel that higher power to create miracles?

It has often been said that there are only two ways to live your life. One is as though nothing is a miracle. The other is as though everything is a miracle.

I agree with the latter. Making miracles is a matter of binding our consciousness with Universal consciousness. We may not be in command of our miracle-making potential at the moment, but that's because we've been culturally programmed to dwell in an automated, unconscious, and marginalized state of realization.

We have been trained to exist in an ethos of unconsciousness that has fed the great myth of the limited self. We have been taught to believe we are confined and bound by extreme limitations because we exist in a three-dimensional world. The result of this education creates an identity crisis of epic proportions that we all suffer from because we accept it as fact. By recognizing that we are unlimited, we have the ability to transform beyond this absolute misidentification of self so that we can achieve our miracle-making potential.

We *are* imminently more powerful than we've been led to believe. Our fully realized being-ness represents higher states of consciousness than we may be familiar with, but we can shift the ethos—the culture—to accept that we *are* superconscious beings who possess the potential to make miracles. Combining our highest level of personal consciousness with that of the Universal mind results in a collective unified field of awareness. It's much larger than personal perception. It is the reality whereby miracles can be performed.

Dispelling the illusion of our perceived limitations begins by acknowledging who and what we really are in our totality. We are much more than a name, a face, and a personality. We are an infinite mind, a fathomless heart, an eternal soul, and an imperishable spirit. We are consciousness that is intended to merge into the greater collective Universal field and destined to evolve into a state of miracle-making superconsciousness.

Rejecting Miracles

I believe the gift of miracles continues to elude us because we've been indoctrinated to accept the boundaries of an ego-based, five-sensory, three-dimensional consciousness. We have not been encouraged to reach for and grasp the prospect of such expanded thought. When it comes to the matter of believing in and performing miracles, we're ill-equipped. We need knowledge and support that the ethos of our culture does not provide. Our rejection of our capacity to manifest miracles doesn't make anybody wrong. It simply suggests that the proper tools and skills to engage the task have not been provided.

We are members of a material experiment. Miracles can and do happen in such a world, but they tend to go unrecognized. We've been indoctrinated to anchor ourselves to a reality baseline, and we dare not stray too far from its core. We reject miracles because the concept can't be allowed in such a physically based realm. In fact, try to hold a conversation with someone about miracles. The possibility is too grand and ethereal to fathom for most to pursue with any sincerity because such a narrow state of conscious awareness simply can't envision such a notion.

How can we change this? How can we overcome our identity crisis and this cultural perception of what we are believed to be? How do we define the complete, immense being that we truly are?

Ultimately, we must heal the contemptuous relationship we've had with ourselves. Our rejection of miracles speaks volumes about our self-restricted doubt. To remedy that, we need to begin by redefining *self,* which includes the realization and acknowledgment of our immortality.

Say I were to ask you, "On a scale from one to ten, what is your miracle-making power?"

What would your answer be?

Most people I've worked with start with a relatively low number on the scale because they've been told they can't create miracles and, therefore, feel incapable.

If we want to thoroughly examine what inhibits our restrictive nature, I suggest we begin by looking at how we measure success. Most of us grew up emulating a vision of success that is achieved by avoiding mistakes.

Achievement by avoidance doesn't allow for any expansion. It nurtures the core identity crisis that we are trying to move beyond. Most of us are extremely capable achievers with a high degree of self-esteem, confidence, determination, and skill. But we've been conditioned to think of ourselves as bound to the limits of material reality, and even the most self-realized among us are inclined to struggle with the concept of making miracles.

When I have posed that question to patients, I'm amazed at how many automatically dismiss the notion that they possess any power, much less the capacity to make miracles. Some simply don't feel deserving enough to wield such immense potential, which underscores a very important point: it's less about the miracle and more about the miracle maker.

It's also less about accepting the prospect of miracles and more about rejecting the great myth of the materially limited self. We are mind, heart, soul, and spirit. Accepting and understanding the total self that we embody releases us to cultivate and engage our miracles.

Accepting Miracles

To take the first step toward accepting the possibility of miracles requires that we cross the line of outright rejection and head in the general direction of a willingness to believe. Acceptance represents a positive, although somewhat passive, stage in our miracle-making evolution. It opens the door of opportunity and is an important step along the way to bigger and better things.

Next, just beyond our willingness to believe, we must engage in action. Rejection has no intention and no action associated with it. Acceptance is the first stage of miracle-making evolution that requires an action.

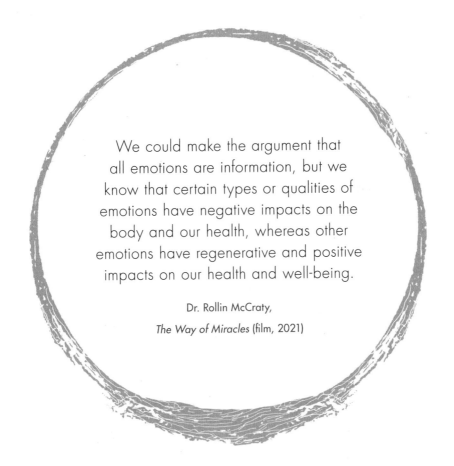

We could make the argument that all emotions are information, but we know that certain types or qualities of emotions have negative impacts on the body and our health, whereas other emotions have regenerative and positive impacts on our health and well-being.

Dr. Rollin McCraty,
The Way of Miracles (film, 2021)

Everything is energy, and thoughts and words represent powerful manifestations of energy. Positive words, like the word *miracle* itself, are not only energizing—they're transforming! The action associated with acceptance begins with the constant presence of positive, empowering words in our self-dialogue.

As Dr. McCraty has stated, affirmations of value begin to change the ethos in which we exist. Evolution of reality starts in the mind with words, visions, and imagination. What if we viewed miracles as untapped energies awaiting our conscious activation? Once that energy is engaged, miracles would begin a fluent process of giving back because every miracle lays the foundation for the next miracle.

Expecting Miracles

Thoughts are things because energy and matter are transferable. Harvard Medical School researcher Robert Rosenthal explored a number of double-blind studies that detailed how expectancy influenced scientific outcomes.[3] We tend to get what we expect, exactly as the science of placebo/nocebo has clearly established. That indicates that expectancy is the energy of intent that manifests in matter.

Neuroscientific research has shown that expectancy alters brain wave patterns via a specific part of the brain called the anterior cingulate cortex. The studies demonstrated that if a person imagined an event with a sense of confident expectancy, the brain produced the exact neurochemistry that it would produce if that person was actually experiencing the physical event. That means that all miracles that ultimately manifest in the physical are initiated by visualized thought.

Another interesting series of studies performed at Harvard Medical School in the 1980s found that when untrained musicians simply imagined that they were playing certain assigned piano pieces, they activated the same brain response as the trained virtuosos who actually played the pieces.

Visions initiate the process of birthing new realities—the energy of thought transforms it into matter.

When imagination meets expectancy, miracles begin!

Though it may seem that these manifestations come from what might appear to be nothing more than the ether of imagination, this is actually where the energetic properties of thought begin to form reality. But in order to move in the direction of creating reality, we must first acknowledge that expectancy is empowered by the willingness to believe.

Belief represents raw power. It not only generates energy—it also produces a demonstrable change in physical reality. Ongoing research continues to show that our cells receive and process information transferred through thought, which indicates that genes and DNA do not control our biology. It appears that our DNA is controlled by our thoughts and subtle intentions that originate from outside the cell.

Our thoughts alone have the power to affect our physical and mental reality. Expectancy enables us to access our unlimited power. Belief in and expectancy of miracle-making power actually generate it.

Making Miracles

The step beyond believing in and expecting miracles is to create them. If expectancy initiates the material production phase of miracles, then visualization, or visual creation, as I like to call it, is an action step that can produce mass production. As powerful as expectancy is, it still has a tinge of passivity. Expectancy represents positive, mental intent where the next step of visual creation represents active demonstration.

The creational power of visualization has been studied extensively for decades. What these studies have all clearly established is that "seeing is believing," even if envisioned only in our consciousness. The other half of this equation is perhaps best summarized by author Wayne Dyer who said, "Believing is seeing!"[4]

There was a series of fascinating visualization studies that were published in the December 3, 2009, issue of *Psychology Today*.[5] One of the studies looked at the brain wave patterns of weight lifters. It cited that the more the weight lifters visualized lifting heavy weight, the more likely they were to improve their ability to physically perform.

This is the response to thought in specific areas of the brain that dramatically affect physiology. In fact, the authors of these studies agree that mental practices are almost as effective as physical practices, and combining the two is more effective than doing either one independently.

In a similar study, Cleveland Clinic's exercise physiologist Guang Yue worked with a team of researchers to compare subjects that worked out in a gym with those who simply visualized the same workouts.[6] Yue found a 30 percent increase in muscle strength with those who went to the gym and a 14 percent increase with the group who merely imagined or visualized doing the same exercise routine. This remarkable data demonstrates that the energy of thought, coupled with active visualization, produced a material response that is equal to approximately half of what was achieved through physical effort.

Thus, the brain initiates the process of miracle-making reality from what we originate as an image in our mind. Our brain is truly capable of producing the same neurological response to imagined events that it does to those that are materially performed. Whether we are playing the piano or simply imagining it, our brain registers the concept and relays it to the rest of our entire being with equal intensity. That means that what we produce via envisioned thought becomes deeply and instantly rooted in the reality machinery of our brain. It seems our brain was designed to support the process of giving birth to miracles by feeding them imaginative thoughts.

Our Miracle-Making Self

We're made up of two distinctly different selves and each of those imparts very different stories about who we are. One self, the material self, generates its own finite field. That field is restricted by the dictates and limitations of time and space. Miracle making is generally not possible in such a finite, material field.

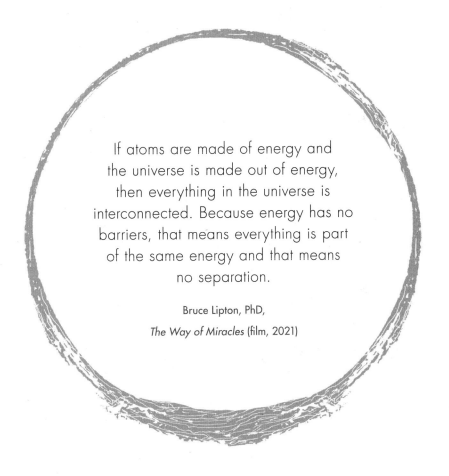

If atoms are made of energy and the universe is made out of energy, then everything in the universe is interconnected. Because energy has no barriers, that means everything is part of the same energy and that means no separation.

Bruce Lipton, PhD,
The Way of Miracles (film, 2021)

Our other self is boundless. It is part of the infinite Universal field of superconsciousness. This is a field that is unlimited. It is where miracles are bountiful.

We are all miracle makers. But in order for our miracle-making power to manifest, we must first identify with and, ultimately, exist within and emanate from that boundless self, which draws unlimited power from the infinite Universal field.

The real challenge facing us is that we are part of a dualistic Universe. While everything is unified, it also has a dual nature. All things, including you and me, are composed of energy and matter, spirit and body, and soul and ego. To add to this challenge, we are part of a cultural experiment whose ethos is profoundly biased in matter, physical form, and ego. Our basic survival may depend on material, physical, and ego consciousness, but our miracle-making capability requires energy, spirit, soul, and ultimately, superconsciousness.

It's about the consciousness we cultivate. This is key. By increasingly turning our attention to prayer, meditation, and spiritual contemplation, we elevate the energetic frequency of our consciousness. In turn, those actions increase the opportunity to identify with and emanate from our boundless miracle-making self.

It is through the refinement of our consciousness that we develop a greater understanding about the true nature of our power.

Because of our material, physical, and ego bias, we're accustomed to mistaking blunt force for power. However, power is very subtle in the realm of energy, spirit, and soul. In fact, the more subtle the energy is, the greater its power. It's a reality where less is more. It seems a bit of a paradox, a sort of drawstring effect: the weaker the material properties, the stronger the energetic properties. Perhaps it's best exemplified by the energetic medicine known as homeopathy. Homeopathic medicine is similar to the concept of a vaccination, as it introduces the body to a very small dose of a toxic agent. The purpose is to direct the body's immunological attention to any possible exposure. The difference is that in homeopathy, the exposure is no longer composed of a material dose because it's diluted down to the remaining energy of molecular memory. The more diluted the material properties, the stronger the energetic properties of the medicine.

So, as matter becomes lesser, energy becomes greater, and so it is with us. As our material force contracts, our miracle-making power expands.

We must never forget that we are not merely makers of miracles; we are miracles. The river of creation flows both from us, as well as to us. Power represents the eternal spark that enlivens the continuum of creation. And as much as we may be reluctant to admit it, we are Divine. Our boundless presence knows no end, nor can it ever be repressed by the limitations of what we think of as mortality. It's not just all right to marry our mortal self with our immortal self. It's essential. It speaks to the very reason we are consciousness.

In actuality, we can't be any less Divine or any more human than we are. We are a perfectly imperfect dichotomy. In our boundlessness, we are unified with our human nature. In our finiteness, we are consolidated with our Divine nature.

The important question here is, Can our two divergent natures live in a miracle-making harmony with each other?

The good news is that there is a bit of wizard in all of us. Over the centuries, organized religion has done great damage to that wizard. Rather than accepting miracle making as an expansion of consciousness that merged our higher awareness with God's mind, it cloaked its beauty in evil, dark forces, judgment, and persecution. Calvinism spawned a misconception that we are all guilty sinners who, because of our sinful nature, are disqualified from miracle making, proclaiming that only the unblemished have access to the righteous power to perform miracles.

Oddly, the essence of our miracle healing power can be found in a seminal discussion about our duality. With superconsciousness, our mortal awareness merges with transcendent Universal consciousness, revealing that we are both human and Divine. In the superconscious state, we understand ourselves as both saint and sinner and therefore have the potential to forgive ourselves of our own sinful nature. This is the solidarity of our two selves, the material self and the boundless self, from which miracles emerge.

Cultivating Miracle-Making Power

The Universe isn't merely a vast, cold, inanimate place that's part of a definition of space. The Universe is more like a living being, no different than you or me. It's an energetic being with a pulse, a heart, a soul, and a spirit. It feels, it needs, it loves, and it deeply appreciates any and all heartfelt currents of care and compassion that are directed its way. If we want to access our superconscious miracle-making power, we need to shrink the concept of the Universe down to a lovable size, so that we can wrap our arms around it and embrace it.

Do you have a relationship with the Universe? Is it of a loving nature? Is it personal?

We have been taught to pray "to that," which we are led to believe is greater than us. In our prayers, we "ask for," with no consideration of ever giving anything back in return. We are not inclined to consider the perspective of such a relationship. But we are also mistakenly led to believe that such Divine Universal energy is separate from us. Due to its power and vastness, it couldn't possibly need anything from us. Right?

What if we were to alter that notion and were to develop a reciprocal relationship with the Universe, a relationship that was loving and personal? It may be difficult to envision such a possibility. But by attempting to consciously develop an intimate relationship with the Universe, we will engage the process of cultivating superconscious power.

If the power of making miracles is what we want to achieve, we might consider praying *for*, rather than *to*, the Universe. Why is the word *for* important? Because by praying for, communicating with, caring about, and giving our love to the Universe, we become an integral part of the ultimate miracle-making story that encompasses all that exists. The Universe is complete; the only thing it can't get enough of is love.

There's a simple formula at work here. It's a formula that will shift your present precepts and views from one of destruction to one of creation. In short: Give your unbridled love to the Universe and become the miracle that makes miracles. As your expression of love for the Universe grows, your ability to experience the blessings of miracles will increase proportionately. It's as simple as that.

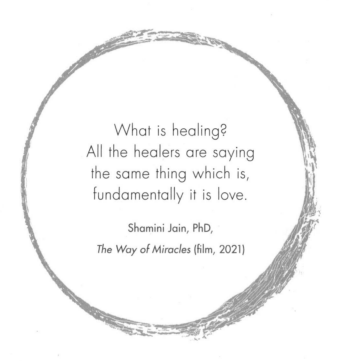

What is healing?
All the healers are saying
the same thing which is,
fundamentally it is love.

Shamini Jain, PhD,
The Way of Miracles (film, 2021)

The Superconscious Power of Unconditional Gratitude

The word *gratitude* has a strong spiritual meaning yet, ironically, our most common translation of the word is rooted in materialism. While it's true that it suggests a deep sense of appreciation, it's usually appreciation of some form of material that one has been given. Generally, we think that without the receipt of something, there is no need for gratitude. That perspective is misaligned with superconsciousness, because pure gratitude is unconditional. We don't need a physical object to spark gratitude; it should be all-encompassing.

We've been taught that when one receives or something good happens, the recipient is grateful. But when bad things happen to us, there's no need for gratitude.

Superconsciousness is aligned with the Universal aggregate that implies both unconditional and undivided wholeness. Good and bad are inseparably interdependent parts of one whole.

Superconsciousness understands that there's an important distinction to be made between unconditional and conditional gratitude. Unconditional gratitude represents one of the very highest energetic frequencies.

Conditional gratitude is more of an emotional response than a state of being, and it doesn't hold the same transformative power. Conditional gratitude cannot be considered an action because it's a reaction to the receipt of some form of gift or blessing. While conditional gratitude is a beautiful expression, unconditional gratitude is a state that is whole and complete. It's not a reaction, and it's not dependent upon an initiating form of action.

Rather than being about feeling blessed, unconditional gratitude is more about becoming a blessing, more about giving than receiving. The more we become one with this elevated state of consciousness, the more we become the gift. This pure state of gratitude is the joy of becoming the gift.

The whole point of attaining superconsciousness is to spiritually evolve and to expand our transformative power. If there is no gratitude, there isn't an impetus for spiritual evolution or transformative power.

Think of a time when you felt an amazing sense of appreciation and gratitude for just being. Feel into that time when you experienced the is-ness of being present within your own subjective and objective reality. The transpersonal self gives the ultimate gift of enlightenment to the personal self. That means that we are both giver and receiver. We become the circle of energy that gives and receives equally because unconditional gratitude between the subjective and the objective creates a natural energetic attraction.

Imagine a vulnerable part of yourself that deeply appreciated a powerful part of yourself or vice versa. You are bringing the whole of your being together. The state of appreciation that exists within each and every one of us is permanent and doesn't require conditions or prerequisites to be present. Recognition of that is the superconscious power of unconditional gratitude.

The Superconscious Power of Lucid Stillness

States of consciousness generate powerful fields of energy. They can evolve into profoundly healing or dis-easing thoughts and emotions. Acute or chronically negative thoughts and emotions are potentially destructive. They can dangerously disturb the delicate equilibrium of our wholistic balance. Negative emotions should not be underestimated, as the destructive potential of a single negative emotion can be indelible. From a conscious perspective, things like jealousy or rage can alter our fate in an instant.

Those are all reasons that I believe we must nurture ourselves with more positive, uplifting internal dialogue. But superconsciousness can help us transform our destructive states by exercising the power of lucid stillness to snap out of and ultimately heal ourselves from this dis-easing process.

Lucid stillness is a natural byproduct of superconsciousness. We can choose to drop out of a negative state by mastering the moment with mindfulness and the power of lucid stillness.

The word *lucid* is recognized in a literary sense as "luminescent" or "light emitting." *Stillness* may be best described as "absolute serenity." Therefore, *lucid stillness* might be defined as "light-filled serenity." Unlike the plethora of destructive states characterized by restlessness and confusion, lucid stillness is the only state generated by superconsciousness. It's a state of tranquility reflecting both the light of our consciousness as well as the Divine light of Universal consciousness. Taking the quantum leap from the destructive to the superconscious state represents the never-ending journey of a single step, from the monkey mind, unsettled and confused, to the Divine mind, which is whole and fulfilled.

The Divine mind shines through all. Our soul, the source of our being, is a microcosm of the light just as the Universe is a macrocosm of the light. Through lucid stillness, the two beams of light become fixed on each other, and at that point superconsciousness radiates its miracle-making incandescence.

While there is no question that practices like meditation, deep relaxation, and trance states can assist with superconscious evolution, superconscious healing requires the cultivation of sustainable lucid stillness with our every action. It's only when we develop the ability to master the art of being in the midst of all our doing that we truly enter into the realm of superconsciousness.

Literally every patient I have worked with was somewhat aware of the subtle, dis-easing roots of their illnesses. Many were aware that they'd become victims of a tragic story that they'd unconsciously authored. Their narrative of pain and suffering was disruptive and, in many ways, enslaving. They described disconcerting thoughts that came at them in endless waves with an unrelenting, and at times overwhelming, force. Many also learned that the force of such darkness could never stand up to the power of lucid stillness.

Committing ourselves to sustained states of lucid stillness represents the greatest miracle manifestation of superconscious healing. Think of it as the first medicine because it is the medicine that transforms through the infinite power of peace. Lucid stillness creates peace that comes in a moment and lasts an eternity.

Superconscious Soul Parenting

Superconscious healing is deeply rooted in the concept of spiritual autonomy. Spiritual autonomy is the greatest power associated with wholeness, especially when we consider that soul is the most preeminent aspect of our wholeness. Simply stated, soul is the source of our being and therefore our greatest power.

I recently enjoyed a follow-up office visit with a fifty-year-old woman who first came to see me four years ago. She had previously been diagnosed with stage-four breast cancer. Our visit was a true celebration, as her oncologists recently pronounced her cancer free.

I made it a point to congratulate her remarkable effort. She beat the disease through nutritional discipline and superconscious transformation. Amazingly, she had evolved from a state of absolute fear to a transcendent state of peace and confidence. Looking back on our work together, she recalled one session that she felt made a profound difference. At the time of the appointment, she was extremely anxious and was so crippled with fear that she was unable to fully function. She recalled that I had encouraged her to engage with her *superconscious soul parent.*

I explained to her that during our childhood years, we all experience forms of irritation during periods of acute stress. They remain embedded in our unconscious mind. I told her that these "frozen" states are neurobiologically retained within our bodies, and they are reexperienced whenever similar emotions are stirred up later in life. As a result, grown adults are often neurologically reduced to their frightened child self.

I told her that while in spirit, between lifetimes, we choose our parents. We make that selection because only their specific flaws will bring about the necessary painful lessons that will ultimately inspire us to spiritually parent ourselves. I reminded her that her parents' failings were exactly what she needed to awaken her personal superconscious soul parent's love and guidance in all the ways that her earthly parents could not.

I told her that there are many important secondary reasons why we've come into this existence, but one of the primary reasons is to engage the love and guidance of our superconscious soul parent. To put it another way, it allows us to autonomously parent ourselves. Each of us has a fair amount of superconscious soul parenting that we came in to accomplish.

Remember that we are composed of two distinctly different selves: a mortal self, the ego, and an immortal self, the soul. Our mortal self is temporary. It is flawed and vulnerable. Our immortal self is eternal. It is perfect and omnipotent. Within the vast unconscious depths of our mortal self, we contain an archive of karmic suffering. These are painful life lessons that result in a relentless drive to escape, avoid, and deaden the pain. Unfortunately, there is no escaping. Our mortal self is its own perpetual source of pain and suffering. The result is that our mortal self is drawn to the distraction of pleasure in a myriad of forms that produce in an endless loop of afflictions and addictions.

The unconscious mortal self is the vehicle of karma or lessons, while the superconscious soul self is our vehicle of transformation. The superconscious soul parenting process is difficult, but the Universe has provided some fail-safes to help lighten our load. An important safety measure is that perfection and imperfection are intertwined. Nothing goes to waste in the Universe. An opportune way to view this is that imperfection ultimately flows into the vastness of perfection. As in the placebo effect, much of what we believe does indeed happen to us and happen for us. Every karmic lesson inevitably brings us closer to moksha, to liberation.

Thus, there is symmetry between karma and moksha that can be accepted and understood by an enlightened mind. Notice how I preceded the word *understood* with the word *accepted*? That's because enlightenment awakens within us only after we've surrendered.

We need to learn how to surrender and let go of all blame and resentment that we've erroneously associated with our imperfect, mortal parents and, for that matter, all our karmic relationships. Then the perfectly symmetrical physics of moksha allow us to become everything to ourselves. We ultimately become the parents to ourselves that our worldly parents couldn't be. Remember: we choose our parents. They are part of our lives to fulfill our choices of lessons and to allow us to be our own parent to ourselves so that we may heal on many levels.

The Razor's Edge of the Superconsciousness

Superconsciousness represents a quantum leap in the direction of enlightenment, but it's important to be aware that sometimes insight can be accompanied by intense anguish. Discomfort often accompanies the dismantling of an accepted perception. The shift in perception of a previous truth to a deeper identity of it generally is uncomfortable. That serves a great purpose though as it permits us to restructure our conscious intent and identity.

The noted spiritual teacher Adyashanti perhaps put it best when he said, "Make no mistake about it, enlightenment is a destructive process. It has nothing to do with becoming better or being more or less happy. Enlightenment is the crumbling away of untruth. It's seeing through the facade of pretense. It's the complete eradication of everything we imagined to be true."[7]

The result of such a transformative process is inclined to bring about a healing crisis. The more superconsciously refined our energy development, the more hypersensitive we become to the blinding darkness of the world.

As our consciousness becomes more expansive and aware, we tend to become more susceptible to both our internal energies as well as our external energies that surround us. Intentions, thoughts, feelings, memories, dreams, people, food, noise, environments, conditions, and circumstances of all kinds are likely to have a more pronounced effect on us. That's because as we evolve in superconsciousness and refine our vibration to it, our tolerance of unrefined energy greatly diminishes.

The people we surround ourselves with, the food we eat, and the actions we engage in must all vibrate at a higher frequency or they don't feel like they fit in our lives. Also, as our vibrational frequencies rise, we may find ourselves radically changed in a way that craves peace and quiet refinement.

Though we're temporarily *in* the world as superconscious aspirants, we must learn to identify ourselves as being eternally *of* the Universe. By identifying and ultimately grounding ourselves in our Universal identity, we provide ourselves with substantial insulation from the world's exterior noise and destabilizing forces.

The material providence that appears to surround us is but an illusion. It's not about being fulfilled by the illusion of the exterior world; it's about being filled full by the eternal source within.

Superconscious transformation is difficult. It brings about the death of illusions we have identified with and forces us to realize that we can never again revert to our former self. There is only one way. We must move forward on the razor's edge of a tightrope on the sacred journey to superconsciousness.

Observing Yourself Exercise

After you finish reading this chapter, put down your book for a moment and find your way to the nearest mirror.

Look into the mirror. Fix your gaze on the innermost center of your eyes. What do you see?

While your reflection peers back at you, I'd like you to ask yourself who you really are.

Can you feel your mortal self being observed by your immortal self?

Are you the observed and the observer?

Can you feel the connection?

If you can, you are witnessing the conscious soul that you are.

One purpose of this exercise is to inspire some self-consciousness.

I use the hyphenated term *self-consciousness* in a more vast way than the normal understanding. We typically associate the concept of *self* as an objective perspective. Rarely do we occupy self from both an objective and a subjective vantage point, as you did by looking at yourself in the mirror.

By objectively and subjectively observing the essence of your being-ness, you can't help but become more attuned to the presence of your soul.

The underlying intention of the observer exercise is to initiate deeper thoughts about perception, identity, and consciousness by inspiring a moment's recognition of the pure awareness that you are!

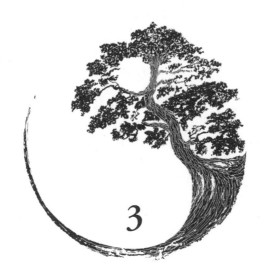

3

States

As a noun, the word *state* refers to a condition, quality, or the status of something, or in our case, someone. When we address the state of a person's consciousness, we're generally speaking about their frame of mind, their emotional being, their attitude, and the presence of their awareness.

Our minds are deluged with an endless torrent of thoughts, perceptions, memories, and emotions, all of which contribute to our varying states of consciousness. All our states are interrelated, interdependent, and relevant to our understanding of superconsciousness, for within our deeper states, there is an infinite reservoir of untapped power. We're going to focus on the diversity of our conscious states.

It's the potential power of these states of awareness that have long captured the imagination of those working to achieve superconscious. This was especially true for many of those from the ancient Eastern cultures. Several of their sacred rites and rituals induced meditative and trancelike states. These practices often brought about visions and, when mastered, generated transcendent powers.

The Upanishads are a sacred Hindu treatise that is part of the two hundred ancient Sanskrit texts called the Vedas. These date back to 800 BCE. Sometimes referenced as the highest form of human wisdom, the Vedas contain the seminal spiritual themes shared by Hinduism and Buddhism.[1] These texts were written to reveal the reality of *atman*, which is a Sanskrit word for the ultimate true self . . . the soul.

The ancient Mandukya Upanishads are among the earliest of spiritual wisdoms to advance the position that there are multiple, separate states of consciousness. According to these texts, there are four:

1. Waking (Jagrat)

2. Dreaming (Svapna)

3. Deep Sleep (Sushuputi)

4. Pure Consciousness (Tuiya)

Jagrat is representative of gamma burst brain waves, manifesting as a calm but heightened state of alertness. In the state of jagrat, the vigilant mind and survival brain are one. Here, perception is focused on operating in the physical world in a predominantly sensory, anticipatory manner, but with a calm, purposeful clarity.

In the ancient East, the most important reason for understanding the various states of consciousness was the identification of the ultimate true, eternal self. Jagrat represents a reflection of the predominantly erroneous state of self-identification common to the Western world. The Western perception of self is predominantly based in the material world. In the West, self is representative of body, personality, and ego. In the East, it is believed that in jagrat, one may be very easily deluded into accepting the fleeting material illusion as real.

In svapna, or the dreaming state, the ancients believed that we experience dreams during sleep as well as daydreams, fantasies, memories, and imagination while in the waking state. We enter this state just before falling asleep and just prior to fully awakening. We might do well to think of this state as an alpha brain-wave state, representing the relaxed, meditative mind. It's in this clear, peaceful state where we first catch a glimpse of atman, the soul. Here we can see the doors of higher consciousness opening us up to transcendent power.

Sushuputi is a state of deep sleep, or what sleep specialists term the delta brain-wave state. It's viewed as a more of a pure state of consciousness because it is egoless. We might think of the delta brain-wave state as a reflection of our superconscious mind.

Tuiya is pure consciousness. It might be best conceptualized as a theta brain-wave state where our senses are withdrawn from the external world and singularly focused on signals originating from within. In this state, one can fully recognize the true soul identity.

Remember that most states of consciousness represent both cause and effect. If we experience a bad dream, we typically have a bad day. If we have a bad day, we generally have bad dreams. This is not so with tuiya. The state of tuiya is a pure state, which transcends cause and effect as it presents us with an unobstructed view of atman.

The ancient Eastern cultures identified four states of consciousness. Today, in the modern West, EEG (electroencephalogram) research has confirmed that there are no less than eight brain wave states, or frequencies, that are measured in cycles per second called hertz (Hz). Different frequencies have different effects on the measurement of our brain waves. Various studies have shown that eight distinct states of consciousness resonate to specific groupings of hertz measurements. These are:

1. Beta, 14 to 30 Hz, waking

2. Alpha, 9 to 13 Hz, meditative

3. Delta, 0.5 to 4 Hz, trance

4. Theta, 4 to 8 Hz, pure consciousness

5. Gamma, 30 to 100 Hz, unified consciousness

6. Hyper Gamma, 100 Hz, transcendent consciousness

7. Lambda, 100 to 200 Hz, plenary consciousness

8. Epsilon, 0.5 to 0 Hz, circinate consciousness

The frequencies tend to increase relaxation, awareness, focus, and concentration in ways that enhance and empower the capacity of the mind. Each of these brain wave states provides a specific contribution to the cultivation of superconsciousness. Of these eight, the two states that are best designed to help us access superconsciousness are alpha and delta. It's through alpha meditation and delta trance relaxation that we generate frequencies that can transport our personal consciousness across a virtual bridge to merge with the Universal mind.

While both meditation and trance states are keys, it's important to try to nurture a higher state of mind on a moment-by-moment, day-to-day basis. Meditating for twenty minutes twice a day is a wonderful tool, but we want to change the energetic constitution of our mind and evolve our consciousness in such a way that it *becomes* meditative. It's a matter of taking the energy produced by meditation and disciplining ourselves to renew it, sustain it, and further evolve it until it becomes transcendent energy. We need to learn to adjust our thinking. This energy is more than merely a state of mind that we can visit from time to time. We need to realize this is an elevated consciousness that we can *become*.

Dream States

Dreams are sensorimotor, which means that they involve both sensory and motor functions or pathways of the brain. They often correlate with an ongoing waking narrative; sometimes they inform us of issues we need to look at more closely. The dream state taps into the repressed unconscious mind, and it's a sort of release valve for unconscious memories that might be painful or suffering that we may have experienced. Remember, the subconscious mind forgets, but it doesn't block. The blocking mechanism of the mind is found in the unconscious mind. Dreaming is therefore a state that heals. Renowned Swiss psychiatrist Carl Jung believed that dreams integrate our conscious with our unconscious lives.[2] Through a process Jung called individuation, we have the ability to solve conflicts and discover cures that are hidden deep within us.

Dreams release tension in the form of stories that our brain tells us during sleep. These stories are composed of a collection of memories, emotions, symbols, and images that involuntarily occur during the seven stages of REM (rapid eye movement) sleep, and on average, dreams commonly last anywhere from three seconds to thirty minutes. Dream researchers have discovered tens of thousands of meanings, symbols, and keywords associated with dream interpretation, but it's important to realize that your dream is individually yours.

Dreaming manifests in our deeper levels of consciousness, but for the most part, it takes place in the spiritual realm. Dreams engage our deeper spiritual reality, which enables us to reach higher levels of ethereal awareness. By making that connection, dreams unconsciously and subconsciously open us up to the greater possibilities of the supernatural. Many a miracle is born in the world of dreams.

Imagination States

Reality and imagination stream from the brain in two different directions, but they activate the same pathways. Visual information garnered from real events seen by the eyes is transmitted upward, from the occipital lobe to the parietal lobe of the brain. Imagined images seen by the mind's eye flow downward from the parietal to the occipital. One flows upward, and one flows down, but the result is the same. As described earlier, each stimulates the very same neurological chemistry in the brain no matter if it is visually seen or imagined. Imagination is an empowering higher state. This is why it is so important to cultivate personal power through imagination.

As a parent, I learned to use imaginative creativity to ease certain situations. I maintained a wonderful tradition with all three of my children when they were very young. The great mystery of the darkness of night has always been a source of angst for many children, and mine were no different. So, every night before they went off to sleep, I would think up some parable or symbolic story to distract them from their restlessness and anxiety. I made up some really fun, magical, and spellbinding stories. Every now and then I came up with a real doozy!

Among the stories I remember best was the ongoing account of Smitty, a two-fingered, imaginary being who was always readily available to show up for my kiddos, whenever they needed him most. If they ever struggled to finish their dinner or couldn't sleep at bedtime, Smitty would magically appear to reassure and soothe them. All it took to bring Smitty to life was a little imagination. The kids found great comfort in knowing that they were always an imaginary thought away from being greeted by Smitty and his magical, make-believe presence. Smitty's enchanting persona inspired us to weave an ongoing tapestry of spontaneous tales and gave us an opportunity to utilize our inexhaustible imaginations together as a family.

One of the narratives the children loved revolved around a story about a little boy named Joey. He was lonely, so he made a wish one night before he went to sleep that he would soon find a special friend. Then, remarkably, the very next day, as Joey was walking in the forest, he came upon a truly amazing sight! He discovered a giant Magic Bird!

The Magic Bird was very friendly and invited Joey to hop up on his back so that they could explore the vast reaches of the infinite universe together. Every night before bed, we'd enjoy a new episode of Joey and the Magic Bird. Together we explored the exciting new worlds of the universe that Joey and the Magic Bird visited. These are very special memories for me, and although it may sound strange, the magical imagining was as beneficial for me as it was for the kids.

There's no question that these colorful, richly crafted stories profoundly inspired their imaginations. And I know that those evenings of mystical flights of fantasy made a significant contribution to the remarkable creative manifest masters they've become as young adults.

It's up to each of us to tap into our imaginative self to manifest miracles.

Imagination can foretell the future. Moreover, it reshapes it. Whenever we imagine, we initiate a creational process that has the power to alter reality. That's due to the fact that, just like everything else in the universe, thoughts are energy and matter. The ratio is important: thoughts are 99.999 percent energy and 00.001 percent matter. The education of our material world is why we are more resistant to accepting energy over material as fact.

From an early age, most of us are taught to think of imagination as nothing more than a childish deviation from reality. It is, in fact, the most powerful creator of reality!

Virtually everything that currently exists in the material world started out as a thought. Then, over time, that thought was repeated in what eventually evolved into a powerful stream of consciousness called imagination.

Look at everything around you. Knowing that all of that began as a thought, ask yourself if you underestimate the true power of imagination.

I recall a patient consultation from a few years ago. A husband and wife traveled up from Florida so that, over a two-day period, she could have a series of lengthy appointments with me. Her husband, many years her senior, sat quietly in the back of the room. He had a remarkably peaceful, if not angelic, aura about him. It was so striking, and it kept drawing my attention and distracting me. After about ninety minutes, she requested a bathroom break. As she left the room, he and I started to converse. We talked for a while, one thing led to another, and eventually I learned that he was a Holocaust survivor. He told me that the thing that saved his life was his imagination and that he had consciously assigned all reality over to the power of his imagination. Every moment during that hellish period of his life was steeped in the deepest recesses of his imagination. In order for him to survive, his imagination became his reality.

Science hasn't ignored the imagination. In fact, researchers have extensively studied the potential and the power of the imagination. Studies focus on the brain's imagination center, the anterior cingulate cortex, while others examine the powerful effect of the imagination on the material and the biological. Most of the research reveals that by merely imagining ourselves engaged in some action, like playing the piano, as we discussed before, the exact same neural pathways in the brain become activated as if we were in fact performing the same action. In the worlds of the brain and mind, material reality and imagined reality overlap.

Psychologists Christopher Davoli and Richard Abrams, from Washington University, prepared a recent study that appeared in *Psychological Science*, where they reported that imagination might be more powerful than we think.[3]

The researchers asked a group of students to search a series of visual displays for specific letters that were scattered among other letters that were simply a distraction.

The students were given a monitor and told to identify the letters as quickly as possible and then to press a button when they were finished. All students held the small monitor. One group was asked to imagine that their hands were free and behind their backs, even though they held a monitor in their hands. The other group was told to both hold and imagine holding the monitors.

The students who imagined themselves as free-handed exhibited far greater speed and dexterity. Those who imagined themselves restricted by holding the monitor with both hands were markedly slower and far less efficient at identifying letters.

The experiment takes us back to the concept that everything is energy and energy can be controlled, and even created, by the power of the mind. Quantum mechanics has proven beyond a shadow of a doubt that the physical world is indeed a sea of energy that materializes and dematerializes repeatedly in milliseconds. That type of research has demonstrated that thoughts are responsible for holding the ever-changing material field together in the form of the shapes and objects we perceive. We might equate it to an old television where a cathode tube is energized by a stream of electrons that hit the screen and create the illusion of continually changing form and movement.

Our ultimate catalyst is thought. It continually alters material reality. And this is especially true of the highly charged thought that is called imagination.

Thoughts are composed of light particles that evolve from formlessness into form by converting from energy to electrochemical matter, which simply means that material reality is forever transitioning from the formless into form. That indicates that the greater the energy is, the denser the matter. Imagination is indeed the most highly charged form of thought energy, and if it's repeated, its field will generate enough mass to ultimately manifest as a form. In much the same way, when we generate profoundly inspired, visually graphic thoughts of a completed, supernatural goal, we are able to imagine our miracles into existence.

Imagination occurs on the soul plane, sometimes referred to as the astral plane. Anytime we are lost in imagination, even if only for a moment, we are actually emanating from our soul! It's through the remarkable transformational empowerment of imagination that we're able to create miracles from the soul plane.

A few of my patients have asked if that means that the imagination is actually an astral vehicle that initiates soul travel where our consciousness can gravitate to a higher plane.

I explain that I believe we all soul travel, and even if it's inadvertent, it happens quite frequently. A simple example could be when we gaze out the window of a moving car. Our imagination drifts to an unrelated thought; in that moment, we're actually soul traveling or having an out-of-body experience. *Spacing out* is the term we often associate with such drifting, and it's perfectly appropriate. That's literally what we're doing! But, because we do it unconsciously, without mindful intent, and without transporting our physical form, we are easily convinced that nothing of any real significance is taking place.

Evolving from imagination to astral projection, or soul traveling, empowers us to magnify our energy far beyond the limitation of material boundaries. Miracles demand a much higher vibration than exists on the material plane. So anytime our soul travels to the astral plane, it becomes charged with energy in this domain of higher frequency. A soul that has been invigorated by the oscillations of the astral plane has much greater access to limitless possibilities. Miracles do manifest in the material world, but they are created on planes of higher frequencies.

I first heard of soul travel in the late '60s, when I tuned in to a television interview with Paul Twitchell on *The John Ankerberg Show*. Twitchell was at the time the Living Eck Master and was one of the founders of a religion called Eckankar, which is still thriving today. Eckankar focuses on soul travel for the primary purpose of advancing soul consciousness. During the interview, Twitchell explained that soul travel is extremely safe and very uncomplicated. To reach the astral level, he suggested that you lie down, get comfortable, close your eyes, and direct your innermost core energy through the center of your chest and out through your third eye, which is between the eyebrows. Keep your eyes closed and allow your life force to flow freely to whatever dimensions it may be drawn to. From there on, it's just a matter of enjoying the ride. Due to our matter-centric culture, we're inclined to think that whatever images appear in our mind are nothing more than abstract imaginary daydreams that have no pertinent connection to reality.

I found the Twitchell interview quite fascinating, and the very next day I purchased his book, *The Key to Secret Worlds*.[4] The book contains remarkable details and accounts about soul traveling. More than anything, his book provided me with an understanding of just how ordinary soul travel is and further clarified how confined I was by the material world. It's quite an adventure to realize your soul can travel the universe while you remain firmly grounded in your physical body, and that the images you experience during your outing are, in fact, other planes and dimensions.

The most common questions that come up regarding soul travel are "Why do it?" and "What benefit, if any, might one derive from soul travel?" Eckankar answers those questions. Its doctrine was founded on the principle that by spending more time within the soul and utilizing soul travel, we develop a greater sense of universalism, elevate our consciousness, and become more spiritually awakened. It asserts that soul travel boosts curative energy and healing power and accelerates personal growth and enhances personal power by boosting brain wave states in a way that allows us greater access to realms of higher dimension where miracles are made.

Heartfelt States

Just how mindful is the heart? We know a great deal about the biological heart, but is there an intelligence factor of the heart? Does the heart have the ability to think?

For more than fifty years, medical science has consistently observed profound shifts in the psyches of vast numbers of heart transplant recipients. Strikingly, they seem to reflect the personality of the donor. Some of the things reported by recipients of donor hearts include: dramatic changes in vocabulary, idiomatic expressions, tastes, opinions, and even emotional states.

The book *The Heart's Code*, by neurophysiologist Paul Pearsall, relates a remarkable story about a three-year-old Arab girl who surgically received the heart of an eight-year-old Israeli boy.[5] One day, out of the blue, the young girl asked for a rare type of Jewish candy that neither she nor anyone in her family had ever heard of before. It was a candy that had been a special favorite of the boy who was her donor. Incredible stories such as this serve as a reminder that far beyond the thinking brain, the human heart has an intelligence of its own.

In 1991 noted stress researcher Lew "Doc" Childre founded The HeartMath Research Institute in Boulder City, California. Inspired by the remarkable results of his ongoing mind-body research, Childre began expanding a concept that's come to be known as heart intelligence. Heart intelligence is described as a flow of intuitive awareness, deeper understanding, and inner guidance that we can access when our heart and mind are in electromagnetic *entrainment*, or synchronization. The research is based on nearly thirty years of scientific measurement of the body's electromagnetic rhythms. HeartMath teams have clearly established that sustained positive feelings revolving such things as love, compassion, and care can generate smooth, ordered, sine-like wave patterns, which lead to the state they refer to as *heart-rhythm coherence*. They discovered that heart-rhythm coherence leads to a plethora of powerful, positive physical, mental, and emotional effects.

About the same time Childre founded HeartMath, one of his fellow researchers, Dr. J. Andrew Armour, made a truly astonishing discovery. Armour identified a bundle of conductive nerves in the heart that are called the cardiac intrinsic ganglia. He dubbed them "the little brain of the heart."

HeartMath researchers have since discovered that a great deal of the flow of our sensory traffic originates in our heart's brain. In fact, ongoing research has established that 65 percent of all our sensory awareness moves from the heart's little brain to the big brain. For far too long we've accepted that the big brain in our head is the center of our body's universe. But consider this: the heart's electromagnetic field generates a measurement of fifty thousand femoteslas, while the brain produces ten thousand. In addition, the electric amplitude of the heart is sixty times greater than the brain. The heart's little brain is electrically one hundred times more powerful and five thousand times more magnetically powerful than the big brain!

It is the heart, and not the brain, that is the thinking center of our being!

The brain is the anatomical organ located in the head and, though the mind is nonlocal or virtually everywhere, many current researchers are convinced that a vast majority of the mind is centered in the heart's brain and not the big brain. Think of it . . . You have a brain beating in your chest!

Thanks to researchers like Armour, we've come to recognize the heart as an intelligent, thinking organ that is in constant communication with the entire body. Not only does the heart always know what's going on, it knows it first! Studies conducted at HeartMath between 2004 and 2007 on the electrophysiology of intuition have shown that the heart's brain

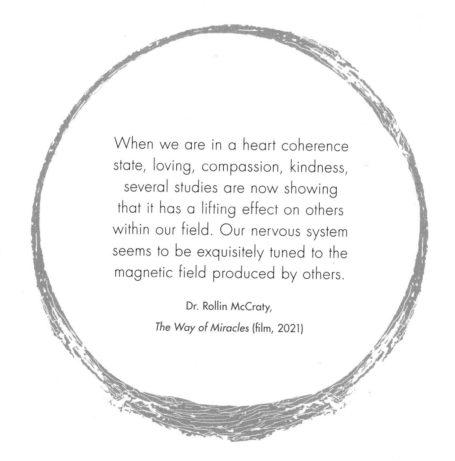

When we are in a heart coherence state, loving, compassion, kindness, several studies are now showing that it has a lifting effect on others within our field. Our nervous system seems to be exquisitely tuned to the magnetic field produced by others.

Dr. Rollin McCraty,
The Way of Miracles (film, 2021)

knows what's about to happen up to a full eight seconds before it does.⁶ And all of this amazing phenomenon is centered in coherency. When our hearts, minds, and emotions are positively in sync, the coherence that results is truly remarkable.

Current HeartMath research is beginning to reveal that there may be a much broader coherency factor that extends beyond the human body. Researchers have discovered that the electromagnetic field of our heart envelops every cell in our body, and it extends far beyond our anatomy, outward into surrounding space, where it interconnects with the universal field.

HeartMath researchers Rollin McCraty, Mike Atkinson, and Jeff Goelitz are currently engaged in research that's referred to as the science of interconnectivity. They've established that when humans generate heart coherence, their electromagnetic field projects with far greater power and at a much greater distance. A much bigger picture is emerging that indicates that by emanating from deeper unifying states of consciousness, we become energetically aligned within the heart and the mind, as well as with the entire living Universe.

This research is employing hard science to validate the coherent interconnectedness of the human self, and the Universe, to demonstrate how they are effectively bound to each other. To understand this, the scientists are examining the energetic connection between all living things. They began the analysis by examining the relationship between human emotions and trees, primarily oaks and redwoods. They discovered that the electromagnetic fields of the trees elicit positive feelings in human beings. That was phase one. Phase two of the research meant they had to take a deeper look at how human emotions affect the electromagnetic fields of trees. To achieve this goal, they applied sensitive electrode sensors to the mighty California oak and redwood trees. The results identified energy patterns that react to human emotions.

As a result of this inquiry, the scientists have discovered that trees possess awareness detectors, proving that the trees have greater perceptive consciousness than ever thought possible. The HeartMath Institute also established that the trees' electromagnetic fields respond differently to the changing circadian rhythms of the sun and moon. Their research continues in order to benefit humans by providing a deeper understanding of how people and trees are energetically connected, gathering information about how trees respond to human emotions generally and how they respond to positive human emotions in particular, and collecting data before earthquakes to aid in prediction and possibly saving lives.[7]

HeartMath research asserts that when our heart, mind, and emotions are synchronized and generating positive feeling states, we unify with the Universal life force. Deeply conscious states that reflect positivity and peace via coherence, meditation, trance, prayer, etc., cultivate a transcendent, unifying energy—the kind of energy that empowers us with miracle-making potential.

Coherence might be more broadly defined as "the formation of a unified whole." The manner in which the whole is unified happens in the flow of the energetic level. The further you investigate nature and the ways of Universal energy, the more you discover the recurring central themes of wholeness and flow.

There is an intrinsic fluidity to the movement of all things in the Universe. The rotational transiting of the planets and stars and the gravitational streaming of running water reveal a powerful dynamic that drives an unceasing natural rhythmic pattern of movement. Only we human beings have inborn free will to defy the fluidity of "the way of things." We have the ability to dance out of rhythm by living at an unnatural pace. I did that and suffered a massive health consequence caused by going too fast and trying to do it all. For us, fluidity should begin as a state—a state that originates in the heart. The coherence that results from our deeper conscious connection to our heart is reflective of our alignment with the universal flow.

The opposite side of the equation, of course, is tension, stress, and beta brain-wave states, which represent our unconscious, and unnatural, rebellion against the flow. This mutiny against the natural energetic flow is the most incompatible and destructive form of our own wholeness. When we consciously flow from the energy of our heart while aligning with positive emotions, we establish coherency within our whole being as well as with the entire Universe. The heart's intelligence can generate a tremendous unifying power, if we let it.

When talking about the power of flow in context with the heart, there's another perspective that is difficult, but very important, to discuss. It's the emotional heart. You'll have to search for quite some time before finding much, if any, information about the emotional heart. Our cultural upbringing has instructed us in a way that has disconnected us from this most vital aspect of self that is so central to our well-being. In fact, I believe our first superconscious priority is to heal our own heart.

We've become tuned out, if not turned off, to our own heart. The success ethic we've been educated in has no tolerance for anything that has greater power than it has. Our system of living has become about quantity, not quality. The quality of emotional life has never been so diminished, and our hearts have never been so disposable. It's one thing that we've been systematically programmed to defend our hearts from each other, but it's quite another that we are now protecting ourselves from our own hearts. It's as if we're holding them in contempt for carrying a pain that we can't seem to escape.

We're raised to survive solely in a physical world. Walk down virtually any big-city street and tell me what you see. Almost everyone appears overprotected and unapproachable. In spite of our obsessive drive toward success, an underlying truth is always going to be how the human heart is affected by the attainment, and the loss, of love. Love is the preeminent sustenance for the human heart. A heart starved for love is simply not sustainable. A heart nourished with love can endure most anything. The heart represents the only aspect of the Source that both literally and figuratively has the power to give and take life.

The time has come for us to reclaim our heart. We want so badly to experience the wholeness of the energy and the wisdom of love that is the heart. We need to learn to be open to the heart's intelligence as it works with the wholeness of the Universe. We can achieve that by living in a place of higher consciousness that will make love eminently more possible.

A Simple Exercise to Balance Your Heart State

HeartMath teaches a simple, but powerful, one-minute technique called Quick Coherence (HeartMath.com/quick-coherence-technique). I use it and have taught it to many highly stressed patients over the years. It never fails to help restore and balance the power of flow to the heart.

Quick Coherence consists of a half dozen slow, deep, five-second breaths that you visually imagine are being inhaled by the heart. As you inhale from your heart, think about someone or something you love very much.

It's truly remarkable how swiftly this exercise generates the power of flow. Feel the flow of the energy it generates and use this technique whenever you feel out of sync.

Love States

The state that speaks to the greatest of all powers is love. And though there is no more powerful energy than that of love, it has never been more misunderstood than it is today. In order for us to become makers of miracles, we must first clarify our understanding of love so that we might become empowered by it.

The process begins with our reidentification of self as soul, heart, and spirit, rather than ego. This initiates our process of overcoming self-contempt and replacing it with self-love. It's much easier to love a soul, a spirit, and/or a heart than it is an ego. Once we shift our identity, we're in a much better position to master self-love. Mastering self-love is the first step to mastering selfless love and, ultimately, enduring love.

Love is not an easy topic to tackle. As it relates to the subject of holistic health and healing, it would seem as though the word *love* would have a significant correlation. After all, it's impossible to be whole and healthy without love, right? Stacked on my shelf are fifteen books that explain how love can make one whole and healthy. I went to the index of each book in search of the word *love*. Not one contained that overused, misunderstood word.

The deeper meaning of the word *love* represents the greatest of all miracles. It signifies a transcendent state of being that produces the very highest of all life-force frequencies. The greatest single factor that influences the quality of life, above and beyond all else, is enduring love. Enduring love is a miracle that makes miracles. Beyond this most powerful form of love, there are many variations.

It's truly astounding how one word can elicit so many different meanings. There's love of God, country, family, and friends. Then there are varying degrees of romantic love, passionate love, and sensual love. There is love of success, material comforts, and money, and the list goes on and on.

The ancient Greeks posited that there are eight principle forms of love:

Eros: erotic love

Philia: affectionate love

Storge: familial love

Ludus: playful love

Mania: obsessive love

Philautia: love of self

Agape: selfless love

Pragma: enduring love

Clearly the beauty and strength of this unequalled, heart-generated power inspired the Greeks to better understand its many magical forms. For our purposes, we are going to focus on the last three forms of love listed: self-love (philautia), selfless love (agape), and enduring love (pragma).

The State of Self-Love

This section on love might well have been positioned under the header of wholeness. Self-love initiates and consummates our wholeness. A self cannot be whole without love. Selfless love cannot be whole without self-love. Self-love is primal. Its presence in one's life is tantamount to autonomy, survival, and prosperity. Although we can't live without it, far too many do, and they suffer mightily as a result.

Over the three and a half decades that I've been a natural healthcare practitioner, I've noted a powerful correlation between self-contempt (the absence of self-love) and dis-ease. In fact, I believe the formula works something like this: self-contempt leads to dis-ease, and dis-ease leads to disease. Because self-contempt is the antithesis of love, it is a principle root cause for the breakdown of body, mind, and spirit. I'm convinced that absolutely nothing disrupts the attainment and sustainability of human wellness more than self-contempt.

Self-contempt is something that I routinely witness in both my work and my personal life. The insidious patterns of self-contempt are rooted deep within the psyche of so many I observe and work with. Self-contempt might manifest as some form of addiction, self-abuse, shame, or even guilt. As long as self-contempt is in the way, the prospect of healing remains at a virtual standstill. I believe the first and most important step to any complete recovery of health begins with the replacement of self-contempt with self-love.

We have two primary lenses of perception through which we view life and formulate the context of our reality. One is our ego lens; the other is the lens of our higher self, or the soul/spirit/heart. Self-contempt can only be seen through the ego lens, which is forever focusing in on all of our human imperfections.

The reason it exists is that it is part of our survival defense system that is in place to prevent potentially life-threatening errors. Call it a critical vigilance. Here, all forms of vulnerable humanness become a liability, as we are continually reminded of all that we lack and, by the process of deduction, don't deserve. With ego, there is little or no sense of deservedness, as even the purity of childhood innocence is all but discounted. When peering through that distorted lens, there appears to be absolutely nothing that is lovable about self. Our accomplishments and material successes end up being interpreted as loveless greed, because we want more, or haunting guilt, because we have too much. Because ego reflects the primary lens that our culture sees through, it represents most of the population. The self-contempt that so many of us suffer from is basically an absence of self-love spiraling out of control.

We each pass through various stages of positive and negative development during our life as we evolve and/or devolve. What we learned in our youth created a foundation for much of the self-contempt that blocks the natural flow of love for self. We were taught to feel good about ourselves when we achieve. It's when we achieve that we're materially rewarded, either by self or by the culture. Material rewards for striving to be better are intended to enable us to develop a sense of pride, or what I believe to be a conditional love of self. We say, "I like me only when I succeed." Such conditioning falls short, for in a competitive culture that programs the masses for human doingness rather than human beingness, there are naturally going to be more have-nots than haves. Winners are rewarded with getting and having. Losers are left to struggle with diminishing self-esteem and the desire to strive for something more. In the end, there remains the burning question as to the true value of what we are striving for.

Many ideas about love and worth have been materially seeded in cultural programming. In the world in which we live, material abundance is directly correlative to simulated self-love. "As long as I can get and have, I can almost feel loved." (Notice I included *almost* in there.) Not getting or having ultimately fuels self-contempt. "If I don't get and have, I don't feel worthy, and because I don't feel worthy, I feel shame."

In today's culture, materialism, or the great golden calf, is in place to serve as a stand-in for self-love. The problem is that there can be no stand-in for self-love. It's a question of intrinsic value. The golden calf can scratch the extrinsic itch on the surface, but it can't reach the itch that exists in the depths of our heart and soul. The price that's demanded is blood, sweat, and tears, but what are we getting in return? Is any of it intrinsically sustainable? If you aren't willing to accept an unsustainable, artificial substitute for self-love, the answer is a resounding no.

Over the years, I've worked with many patients who've attempted to overcome deeply rooted self-contempt issues. From those experiences, I've learned how difficult it is for most of us to be confronted with the challenge of loving ourselves. By the time we reach adulthood, we're so mired in guilt and shame from all the conditional judgment placed on us by society and ourselves that we can't find the handle on self-love. Yet we know that we need to be whole, and to make miracles we must be whole. To be whole, we must master love of self, and that can only be mastered through the higher self.

In the Tai Chi circle, all and everything, including you and me, are part of an endless duality. *Self* represents a myriad of positive and negative energies that add up to one whole being. We are ego and soul. The ego personality does not make it easy to forgive or love. It peers critically at itself through a deeply distorted lens. Therefore, in order to open the door to self-love, we must soften our critical lens of self-perception.

I've discovered that there are two words that soften the critical lens of self-perception and open the door to self-love. The two words are *innocence* and *deservedness*. I often ask patients to rummage through their photo albums at home to search for pictures of themselves as infants and toddlers.

MARK D. MINCOLLA, PhD

I ask them to make copies of the pictures and to post their childhood photos around their home and car and to keep the images in constant view. I then ask them to focus on the pictures and directly associate them with the two words *innocence* and *deservedness*. This exercise ultimately enables them to soften the critical lens of perception and reprogram their consciousness for self-forgiveness.

The next step requires switching lenses of perception all together. The second lens of perception is the lens of higher self. Unlike our ego lens that focuses only on our mortality and our human imperfections, the lens of our higher self sees our immortality, our limitlessness, and our deepest loving nature. When we observe self from this perspective, we are viewing from the vantage of our higher self, and we align with the empowering solidarity of self-love.

So much of the issue surrounding self-love has to do with cultural programming. In the more spiritual Far East, with the influences of Buddhism, Taoism, and Hinduism, cultural programming is generally based on identifying the self as formless and infallible. The higher self is infinite, limitless, and beyond reproach. That makes it much easier to love the higher self than the lower self. More than that, because higher self represents consummate wisdom, it understands that we're complicated beings.

The State of Selfless Love

Self-love naturally flows into the endless river that is selfless love. The selfless giving of love generates an infinite charge of everlasting power. Love from the soul of the self, given unconditionally, produces a powerful energy that vibrates for eternity. Selfless love is truly the gift that keeps on giving, not just for the moment and not just for the recipient. A fulfilled self is free to give from its soul source, without expectations and free from all resentment. Giving is a complete reciprocal act unto itself. There's no distinction to be made between giving and receiving. The key to selfless love's miracle-making power lies with the fact that it is a higher form of giving that automatically gives back; it's unconditional.

Even science is beginning to discover that being in service and selfless giving may, indeed, produce a healing effect on the giver as well as the receiver. Researcher Emily Ansell, of the Yale University School of Medicine, recently reported on a study of hers in *Clinical Psychological Science*. She found that by helping others the effects of stress are dampened. This, some experts believe, might represent an evolutionary rewiring of the human brain.[8]

Previous studies in the field of psychological science indicated that human beings are hardwired for selfishness. But current research is beginning to establish a great deal of evidence to the contrary. They're discovering that we may be changing as a species, and the research indicates that we're developing a more giving and compassionate sense of self in a quest to evolve beyond basic survival. Thus, as our collective consciousness continues to expand, we feel more natural as selfless givers of love. The greater our consciousness is, the greater our sensitivity. The greater our sensitivity is, the greater our natural tendency to open ourselves to the miracle making experience of selfless love.

In my work with patients, I often make it a point to help them experience a selfless love adjustment. I reach far beyond the boundaries of my intellectual mind and channel loving, healing compassion from the innermost recesses of my heart and soul. Sharing my love and energy through meditation that my patients participate in always has a remarkably powerful effect for both my patients and me. In this process, we are giving to each other with a sincere heartfelt openness that raises the consciousness. This type of selfless love adjustment generates such a strong sense of empathy that it generates a compelling frequency that initiates the healing process, which directly speaks to the energy of selfless love. This, I believe, is due to the power of compassion. Compassion is the driving force behind selfless love.

The power of compassion and its potential amplifies deeply within us all. It reflects our most heartfelt sympathy for the "disadvantaged other" and inspires us to be present with loving, life-changing action. Compassion's middle name is service, and its maxim is "There but for the grace of

God go I." This is where love inspires us to take a step beyond the boundaries of self, to the Universal place where the presence of self is reflected in all and everything. It is here that our compassion opens a door of higher consciousness to a place of unification, a place where all is one and separation is but an illusion. It's through the act of giving compassionate, selfless love that we find our way to hallowed ground of actualization deep within the core of our being. It enables us to take our innate place among the brotherhood of humankind. It is in this place of deep loving compassion and dedication to service that we can gain access to infinite power and miracles.

In my book *Whole Health*, I wrote, "Passion is a word that evokes a powerful visceral effect. Since everything is energy, words are, too. They can generate a strong reaction because they carry a parallel frequency of the concept created by our understanding of the word. In essence, word energy is enhanced by mental pictures and imagery generated by a word's meaning. If any word generates energy, it's passion. The word compassion is equally powerful. I've always said that compassion's energy is passion minus the fire."[9]

Beyond the words lies the energy of compassionate passion and its core effect on each of us.

The power of compassion is beyond question. The human brain produces a number of varied brain wave states, many of which are observable. One state, called beta brain-wave burst, is considered the most powerful brain wave state and was previously thought to be untraceable, until it was observed.

Buddhist monks were the test subjects. Scientists placed brain scan electrodes on the monks to track their brain wave state following a deep, compassion-focused meditation. During this meditation, the monks generated the powerful intention of sending selfless, loving compassion and healing energy out into the world, to wherever it was needed most. To the researchers' surprise, they were able to track beta brain-wave bursts for the first time ever.[10] The demonstration by the monks made it clear to the scientists that the focused intention of their compassion could be observed and that the source of the power was not just from compassion but also from the sheer resolve to love and serve. Ultimately, the tenderness of selfless love accounts for its miraculous power.

The State of Enduring Love

Time and space are but an illusion, especially when it comes to enduring love. Enduring love knows no beginning and it knows no end, for enduring love is immortal. With mortal love, the material illusion of time and space has a bearing in physical reality. People meet, marry, and celebrate anniversaries and divorce in accordance with specific dates and times. In that state of being, life takes place within the confines of its own relative vacuum. Mortal love is aligned with, and restricted by, the dictates of gravity. It manifests strictly within the boundaries of a 3D reality. Mortal love is bound to the ever-unfolding moment. Such is not the case with enduring love, for enduring love is timeless.

There are phenomena that completely transcend time, space, and the third-dimensional reality. The energy associated with enduring love is indeed such a phenomenon. We know that energy can neither be created nor be destroyed. It can only be transmuted. Our bodies pass on, but our energy transmutes. Similarly, with enduring love, only the material aspects of the love experience expire. The energy of love can never die; it continues, forever translating into new forms. Thus, enduring love represents undying energy that infinitely transfers into new being-ness. The concept of immortal love energy transferring into new being-ness speaks directly to the issue of past-life relationships.

There is present-life love, and then there is enduring past-life love. Past-life love relationships are very different from all others. With enduring past-life love, there is a rare state of oneness that exists between two inseparable souls. There are often remarkable similarities in thought patterns, habits, and quirks, and there's generally a strong sense of instinctual understanding between the two individuals. They might also experience flashbacks and memories of past incarnations they have shared. Perhaps the most significant factor associated with enduring love is that the enduring lovers keep returning to each other, and in many cases, they seem to feel it and know it immediately.

Years ago I had an office visit with an elderly husband and wife who shared their beautiful enduring love story with me. Maureen and Robert told me that as young children, they grew up and played together in the same Boston neighborhood. They said that their love connection, even as kids, was something very special. As they explained it, they could feel something very unusual existed between them, but neither of them could quite put their finger on what that was. During their teenage years, their relationship started to grow to the next level, and they began to feel a deeper love for each other. Then, just as their love for each other started to blossom, Maureen's family moved to Columbus, Ohio.

The next decade passed; they lost contact with each other. They both said that even during the decade that they were totally separated from each other, the love they felt for each other persisted. In his late twenties, Robert was transferred to Seattle. He moved into an apartment in a Seattle suburb only to discover that Maureen was living right next door! They were wed within a year and have been inseparable ever since.

I have no doubt that Maureen and Robert are enduring lovers who share an enduring love that transcends time and space and defies all rational explanation. I asked them if they believed in past-life love. They did and commented that if any two people could love each other for an eternity, it would surely be them. They acknowledged that there was an unexplainable, magical familiarity that had always existed between them. It had a forever-like quality about it.

The heart, soul, and subconscious mind of enduring lovers may be likened to an infinite archive. Their archives are filled with Akashic records–like memories of a millennia's worth of lives shared and all the love that encompassed. Enduring lovers are a living example of human love's highest potential. The love experiences of these lovers serve as an inspiring testament to all of the world's lovers. They illustrate that the miracle of love is not only possible—it is what we came for.

Enduring love reminds us that real marriage takes place in the eternal recesses of two souls that unite as one. It has nothing to do with egos, legal contracts, and expensive celebrations that far too often end up with divided material properties and child custody issues. If we fail to master self-love and selfless love, we invariably find ourselves having to contend with the pain and confusion of love lost and haunting loneliness. The world has never needed the miracle of enduring love more, which is precisely why the Universe is bringing so many reincarnated, enduring lovers back to each other at this time.

Enduring love represents the highest form of human relationship. It is the perfect combination of self-love and selfless love. It's a four-way marriage between two souls. I'm married to my soul, and I'm married to your soul. You're married to your soul, and you're married to my soul. While enduring love represents a true marriage of souls, it is inspired and initiated by an incredible process of nonverbal communication between two hearts.

Enduring love speaks its own beautiful, secret language. It is a language that many in this world will never understand for it can only be known by the ageless, entwined hearts of two souls united. Unbound by the limitations of time and space, enduring love is engaged and sustained at an extrasensory level. Enduring lovers communicate through each other's energy fields. They engage in nonverbal, heart-to-heart communication long before their physical forms ever come together. Beyond time, space, form, and human incarnation, enduring love forever flourishes in the magical universe of the soul's eternal heart. The reason why enduring lovers feel as though they've known each other forever is because they have. The power of enduring love is infinite.

The Permanent State of Now

Time and space are intellectual abstracts that are intertwined with the most profound meanings of our day-to-day lives. Though they have forever eluded our grasp, they've still managed to remain directly tied to our core experiences of birth, death, and the journey of life in between. And while their significance in our life is undeniable, they remain far too intellectually abstract to develop any spiritual or emotional inspiration.

There's no denying that classical physics and quantum mechanics have brought great insights to the intellectual quandary of time and space. According to classical physics, space-time is a mathematical model that integrates the three dimensions of space and the one dimension of time into a four-dimensional continuum. Quantum physicists have recently determined that *space-time* is defined as a "product of the entanglement between objects." Therefore, space-time is defined by and dependent upon its relationship to surrounding objects. With entanglement, space-time is clearly aligned with the tenets of superconsciousness, as it alludes to a state of wholeness. The depth and dimension that time and space bring to life clearly have underpinnings in spirituality and emotion, but they remain too academically abstract to generate any appreciable degree of inspiration.

What is inspiring is the timeless, spaceless concepts of NOW and FOREVER. The FOREVER state of NOW presents a reality that overflows with superconscious power.

But ours is a dual nature. We are vulnerable, finite matter that faces mortality while we are simultaneously impervious, infinite energy, indifferent to the illusion of time and space. If our version of reality remains predominated by the negative stirrings of the unconscious mind that we limit by time and space, we will remain ensnared in a state of NEVER.

There is only one thing that remains when there is no NOW and FOREVER. That is NEVER. Far too many are dying from the dis-ease that arises from the deception of NEVER. The unconscious mantra that drives the inner dialogue of those addicted to that false promise is: *I NEVER have and perhaps NEVER will obtain the fullness that I so desperately crave, but I will continue to fight for it!*

NOW and FOREVER are not about fighting to obtain fullness. They are about surrendering to the realization that the fullness of our FOR-EVER self exists and that when we infuse each moment of NOW with our FOREVER self, we remain tapped into the exhilarating flow of infinite abundance.

When we remain grounded in a reality that is anchored to infinity, we empower ourselves to tap into the immortal quality that transcends physical life. And if we commit consciousness to the states of NOW for FOREVER, we liberate ourselves from any and all limitations imposed by the material illusion.

What we think, we become. By coming from our immortal self, our soul, we become immortal. By reprogramming and reinforcing our perception of self as an everlasting, whole being, we are ultimately empowered over the illusion of impermanence. There is no greater power available to us than that which results from a base in the states of NOW for FOREVER.

Birthing the awareness of our true, timeless self is just the foundation. The key is to continually re-create a state of NOW by consciously embracing the immortal identity of self.

The grace that accompanies such superconsciousness is both abundant and instantly available, provided we channel it unconditionally, even during the greatest trials of our mortal lifetime.

We're inclined to experience spiritual mood shifts, driven by the ebb and flow of daily life. We remain spiritually inspired as long as negative unconscious challenges don't overpower the conviction of our higher intentions.

NOW and FOREVER changes the spiritual conversation because these absolutes demand we always and unconditionally forge a path straight ahead. Whenever absolutes are present, the benefits are at least equal to the challenges that may arise. NOW and FOREVER may be uncompromising, but they are also infinitely empowering.

We can all go deeper into self. We have access to a wellspring of infinite power that can be reached via the gateway to our soul. We are comprised of the infinite; we belong to the infinite and therefore we are the infinite. Far beyond our ordinary, mortal illusion of self, we are extraordinary. It is the extraordinary self that is designed to perform in the realm of NOW and FOREVER. It is that extraordinary self that is equipped to continuously renew the state of NOW and to fill it with uncompromised consciousness from our FOREVER self.

This is where a perfect symmetry emerges. It's not just about where we emanate from—it's also about who and what we become when we do. By originating in the soul, we are attuned to the powers of NOW and FOREVER, and by that precedent, we automatically emanate from depth of our infinite soul. The spiritual aim and target unite as one.

The State of Pure Presence

Our life on this earthly plane is both precious and fleeting. I have worked with many terminally ill patients over the years, and I've often found myself staring directly into the eyes of mortal desperation. I've heard the anguished pleas of "Help me! Don't let me die!"

The less quantity of physical life we appear to have within our grasp, the more we cherish it. Terminal patients have taught me about the absolute sacredness of life as it begins to depart from us. Every word, every touch, and every breath take on an infinite life of its own and our very presence takes on a different quality. During the final physical moments, we are fully conscious and profoundly present. That makes me wonder how much precious life we waste.

If we're not singularly present, we're never fully alive.

The concept of presence represents life's energy at the very deepest, most intrinsic level. It reflects the degree of aliveness with which we experience our life progression. Our love, our intimacy, our creativity, our successes, and even the lessons of our failures are all profoundly influenced by the depth and dimension of our presence.

Instead of freezing the moment before us, hoping that we can garner a deeper and/or more meaningful experience, we take what we can from the experience and impatiently move on to take whatever superficially comes in the ensuing moments. It seems we are never really where we are. We are always on the next square, distracted by our own fragmented perpetual motion. We're living, but due to our lack of undivided presence, we're not alive.

To be fully alive is to master undivided presence, and the key to mastering undivided presence is to center our consciousness within our breath. I call it learning to live a lifetime within each and every breath, and I mean that literally. We take millions of breaths during our lifetime. How many of the many thousands of breaths that you took yesterday were you conscious of? Is there anything more important than your breath? Were there negative, meaningless thoughts that you focused on more than your life breath? Think of how destabilizing many, if not most thoughts are.

Breath is the ultimate still point. Breath is life. It is also the most fundamental process from which to gather our consciousness and ground the power of our presence. By directing the presence of our awareness deep within the rhythm of our breath, we revive our undivided presence. Committing our focus to such an exercise and by engaging it with repetition, we extend our grasp far beyond the limitations of time and space.

Undivided presence represents an energy field that connotes a powerful, secret quality. It is synonymous with leadership. Those who manifest undivided presence stand out for their innate ability to command attention and inspire commitment. You can feel them as they enter a room. Wherever they go, their energy seems to precede them. But this type of power isn't about doing; it's about being.

Undivided presence is a manifestation of superconsciousness that generates a high frequency field. This field propagates radical transformation without effort. It's not an action field of doing or thinking. It is a non-action field that exists as a conscious state of being. The power of undivided presence comes from non-action. If we are in a conscious state of being, we invite the Universe to fill us with the pure power of undivided presence.

The Liminal State

Scientists have scanned the brains of yogis, monks, renowned artists, and great thinkers and achievers in the hope of gaining insights about liminal consciousness. The word *liminal* comes from the Latin root *limen*, which means "threshold." Liminal consciousness represents energy, which is generated whenever we cross over great thresholds and leave something behind to create something new.

Many Buddhist schools refer to the ultimate liminal energy as the bardo state and is best exemplified in the final threshold or cross-over from mortal to immortal life. They believe that powerful energy generated by liminal consciousness is precisely what provides us with the necessary thrust as we break through the ethereal veil between our mortal to our immortal existence. However, the greatest power of liminal energy is not restricted to our final thrust for liberation from the physical. Liminal power is generated anytime we take a risk or leave something behind for the purpose of creating something new.

More than a willingness to experience something new, liminal consciousness reveals an insatiable hunger to reach beyond our mortal knowledge base. It's about moving from the past into the present where we can manifest the future. Science has discovered that it is liminal consciousness that empowers us to experience the highest levels of true joy, self-awareness, peace, and dynamistic flow through the ups and downs of life. Liminal consciousness represents a maximum ability to create new aspects from those that are waning. It requires bilateral synchronization to be readily achieved.

The human brain has two distinctly different hemispheres. The left hemisphere is predominantly analytical, while the right is more intuitive. Most of us tend to use one hemisphere more than the other. Hemispheric dominance establishes a distinct brain imbalance that exerts a profoundly limiting effect on our liminal mind. According to a great number of studies performed over the past three decades, researchers have discovered time and time again that yogis, monks, great thinkers, inventors, artists, and high achievers tend to employ both brain hemispheres together in unison. Most liminal thinkers, those who embrace change and are not intimidated by the great challenge of leaving something behind, recognize they can create something bold and new.

How do we become liminal thinkers? We must first synchronize both hemispheres of the brain.

We can learn to synchronize the brain's hemispheres to enhance the liminal state. During the waking part of our day, our brain tends to settle somewhere between alpha and beta. During the rest and deep relaxation periods, the brain readily shifts between domains. When we are thoroughly relaxed, the brain passes through the zones between alpha, theta, and delta brain waves. That's when we are most likely to engage in what is called hypnoid dreaming. Hypnagogia is the experience of the transition state between wakefulness and sleep. Hypnopompia is the state of consciousness leading out of sleep. Each of these produces a trancelike state that brings our consciousness directly into liminal entrainment. By visualizing our most desired creative dreams during the fertile period just prior to falling asleep or fully awaking in the morning, we can engage the creational power of liminal consciousness.

The State of Unification

Fulfillment means to be filled full. It is every soul's mission to find eternal fulfillment. And, as odd as it sounds, nothing promotes eternal fulfillment more than perfect emptiness. Superconsciousness is perfect emptiness. It does not reflect our besieged, mortal mind. Alternatively, it represents our highest mind and its unification with the supreme, collective mind of the infinite Universe.

Superconsciousness is unlike any other state because the other four states of mind belong to our mortal nature, but superconsciousness is a pre-existing state of Universal consciousness.

Every living thing has consciousness, and the resulting sea of infinite Universal awareness represents a collective state. Some might even argue that, from the para-psychism perspective, even nonliving things have consciousness, that consciousness is a property, if not the essence, of every-thing in the universe.

To attain to such a realm, we need to master the great paradox of active non-doing. Most of us are raised to be unconscious doers. It's not unusual for us to end up addicted to work and obsessive behaviors in an attempt to attain perfection. We are consciously overactive and feel a need to be perpetually busy doing something. If that isn't happening at any given moment, we feel guilt or humiliation for not achieving. That's what we've been taught is the ultimate goal in life.

What we don't understand is that the less we do, the more we invite the Universe to *do* through us. We must learn to consciously do less, to do less with the distinct purpose of doing less. In making this a conscious goal, we would do less and less until we enter the egoless dimension of no-thing-ness. No-thing-ness works on our behalf to open the door to every-thing-ness from the Universe. This enables us to shift from thought to awareness, from human doing to spiritual being, from being a sub-ject that is observed by the world to being an object that observes all and everything through the eyes of the Universe. This is how we utilize perfect emptiness to traverse from the unconscious to the superconscious state.

Perfect emptiness is the natural result of cultivating a no-mind. The ancient Taoist sages taught that we could attain the highest form of spiritual ascension by practicing Wuxi, deep meditation. Employing Wuxi was said to result in Wuxin, an empty state, or no-mind. This meditation is all about using movement, breath, and sound to help construct an energy bridge of awareness from the heart to the spirit. Similarly, in their practice of martial arts and spiritual meditation, the Buddhists refer to mushin. *Mushin* translates to the "mind without mind." Another similar reference is found with the word *karate*, which means "empty hand." Karate teaches that when our hand is empty, we are in a better position to channel the Divine hand of the Universe. The concepts are the same; superconscious attainment requires that we close the door on our cluttered ego mind that can't grasp the concept of miracle making.

Many Eastern cultural practices, Buddhism, Hinduism, Taoism, are designed around the superconscious, as they are, and always have been, more inclined to transcend the mundane and attain to the extraordinary. Here in the West, we are pretty much raised in conscious, subconscious, and unconscious states. That's largely due to the fact that our cultural ways are pretty much driven by free enterprise. It all depends on what kind of life goals one is inclined to embrace. Conscious, subconscious, and unconscious dominance may earn you a stable weekly paycheck, but they're not likely to buy you a miracle.

I've seen a great many of my patients struggle with this dichotomy, and I've seen distinct patterns. Those who strive the hardest to cultivate a transcendent mind clearly have the greatest success at creating healing miracles. Many of them adopt a magical quality predominated by what I call *transpectancy*, or transformational expectancy. They are certain that something truly unique is going to happen to and through them. I've seen these patients generate miracle results, and in many cases against very long odds. In fact, many of my earlier exceptional patients, whom I often refer to as my teachers, inspired me to get on board and to take a much more active role in setting the tone for miracles. By motivationally encouraging them to stick to their all-important plan, I've witnessed the value of engaging with and exciting the spirit. I learned to be careful not to interject from a state of doubt or question. Because my patients were such wonderful teachers, I've incorporated superconsciousness as almost a Divine source of fuel injection for all I come in contact with and for myself.

A particular patient was diagnosed with stage-four breast cancer. At the time of our initial meeting, she didn't strike me as being a very religious person, but the challenge of her ordeal seemed to inspire a very powerful spiritual persona to rise up within her. I've seen many cases like hers where severely debilitated and terminally ill patients experience a profound transformational shift. I have observed and learned that when it comes to making our miracles manifest, it is just as important to become meditative as it is to engage in frequent meditation and trance states. It's about what I call *transformaction* (transformational activation), turning up the energy on whatever turns "the real you" on. There is a significantly more elevated, superconscious version of self within us all. Crisis tends to wake it up. Oncologists ultimately pronounced the woman cancer free. On our last day working together, she broke into tears of joy. Just before leaving, she turned to me and said, "I thank God for the cancer that came into my life to teach me who I truly am."

Healing Our Negative States

The human mind's ability to generate thought and emotion is limitless. In fact, we have the capacity to enter a virtual infinity of mental states. However, our states are most generally driven by our five primary emotions: anger, fear, anxiety, joy, and sadness, even though others exist. Externally reactive states may be natural during childhood, but even as adults, we remain trapped in a maze of reaction. That makes it almost virtually impossible for us to live empowered lives, establish healthy relationships, and escape the ravages of dis-ease. As adults, it's important that we move beyond our childish reactive states and evolve from the vulnerability of unconsciousness to the power of superconsciousness.

Superconscious healing of the mind begins with the cultivation of awareness over thought. Thought emanates from the mortal self; awareness arises from our immortal source. Awareness isn't qualitative or judgmental; it's a reflection of pure observation. By cultivating a greater presence of awareness, we unshackle ourselves from chronic, negative reaction. It takes more than meditation. It's about becoming meditative, about creating superconscious states.

By increasing our pure awareness, we are better equipped to make our state of consciousness a matter of conscious choice. Most of us drift unconsciously through life braced and anticipating life to present us with scenarios that prompt us to react with corresponding emotions. It's all very conditional. Someone, or something, comes into our life that's positive, and we enter into a positive state. If an influence that enters our life is negative, so too is our reactive state.

We hold the ultimate power to make choices. Consciously choosing a positive state before we even get out of bed in the morning sets the tone of the day. Once the choice is made, it's a matter of holding on to the chosen states and not allowing negative influences to weaken your decision.

I often ask those who are stuck in negative states if they've given any thought as to what state they would like to be in. To get out of a negative state, you've got to first understand that you've allowed someone or something to draw you into the negative. Before you can move in a different direction, you must have an idea as to what you'd like to replace it with. It's a matter of choice. It's about choosing the power of conscious action. By choosing superconscious or meditative states of awareness such as calmness and inner clarity, we can birth a personal reality of true power.

Negative unconscious reaction results in distorted dis-ease states that bind us in artificial realities over which we have no power. Many of us are unconsciously authoring the myth of our own demise. Reality is mind driven, and the mind is state driven. If we don't control our conscious states, our states will control us. The tricky part of this is that negative states are emotion based, and emotions are among the most powerful of human forces.

Until recently, it was thought that there were five basic human emotions, but according to a 2017 study published in the *Proceedings of the National Academy of Sciences*, there are twenty-seven human emotions.[11] They are: admiration, adoration, aesthetic appreciation, amusement, anxiety, awe, awkwardness, boredom, calmness, confusion, craving, disgust, empathetic pain, entrancement, envy, excitement, fear, horror, interest, joy, nostalgia, romance, sadness, satisfaction, sexual desire, sympathy, and triumph.

Every one of these emotions represents a force of pleasure or pain. There is no question about the hold that pleasure and pain have over the human condition. Pleasure and pain are the most powerful of all human motivators.

Freud's pleasure-pain principle states that human beings all have an instinctual drive to seek pleasure and to avoid pain, in order to satisfy our basic biological and psychological needs.[12] The central point is that if we are interested in mastering our states, we have to pull a trump card. There is no question that emotion represents a great force, but we must keep in mind that all emotion is reflective of the conscious, the subconscious, and the unconscious. Greater still is the power of the superconscious.

The conscious, unconscious, and subconscious are representative of our human mind. The superconscious, however, reflects the Universal mind. Only the Universal superconscious mind has the power to interrupt a lifelong unconsciously programmed negative state. There are a host of irritating people, places, and things in every life. They seem to be able to effortlessly access and push our response buttons. In an instant, they're able to set us off emotionally. Disturbances like that generate beta brain waves, and beta brain waves are simply no match for the delta and theta brain waves that we produce in the superconscious state.

Enlightening Our Dark States

States may be described as mental climates that we settle into until they become routine. During the average day, we generate numerous shifting states, which are predominantly affected by emotions, some of which are positive and some of which are negative. Our negative mental and emotional states have the power to adversely affect our physical state. In fact, the most commonly occurring negative state we experience is the root source of chronic dis-ease.

Dis-ease is a word that clearly defines itself. It reflects turmoil that festers deep within, disturbing and haunting the mind and spirit to such an extent that it can psychosomatically manifest as physical illness. This type of generated dis-ease and its disabling symptoms reflect an absence of personal power. Wherever there is state-generated dis-ease, there can be no true sense of wholeness or wellness. As long as we remain mired in chronic fatigue producing states that lack peace and solidarity, our spirit will remain too agitated to inspire the making of miracles.

The negative unconscious state represents an archive of suffering. It's a repository of all our blocked and negative memories. It's where pain is barricaded from our reality. It's the domain where much of our dis-ease is rooted. The term *negative unconscious* is a redundancy. The unconscious mind is where we forget because to remember would awaken our buried pain. This is arguably the most important place to direct initial superconscious healing efforts. Here, disturbances from our intentionally forgotten past are the source of most of our disempowerment. Our behaviors, our life decisions, and our relationships are all profoundly affected by the mental climate imposed by our negative unconscious.

Negative unconscious recognition and programming are initiated in the womb and advance during infancy and early childhood. The emotional dynamics of our natal family system have a very powerful influence over our earliest mental and emotional development. During this vulnerable time in our lives, we are 100 percent externally reactive. We learn to assign power to something exterior, without knowing the power that resides within. Soon we become reactive to all those powers that surround us. The only internal proactive power we have is crying out to the world to get our basic needs met. This is the time in our development when we first begin to cultivate and reinforce our chronic reactive states. Unfortunately, as we age, many of us remain unconsciously locked into these power-sapping states. To make it worse, we mistakenly adopt many of the accompanying distortions as reality. For many of us, this represents a crippling adoption process that follows us from the cradle to the grave.

Our distorted reality is often shaped by the toxic influences of those who are closest to us. An unaffectionate father can make a child feel shamefully undeserving of love. Self-blame can, in turn, drive that child to become a dysfunctional perfectionist as they attempt to overcompensate to earn their parent's love. This scenario can easily result in a deep pain that perpetuates throughout an entire lifetime. And such futile striving is likely to be an indirect cause of negative unconscious state development.

Many a child bears witness to tensions between their parents, tensions that generate states of insecurity, fear, and sadness that end up depositing in the archive of the negative unconscious. These reactive, negative unconscious states have the power to distort personal relationships for a lifetime. Observing the chronic dysfunctional dance between our parents can, in many cases, unconsciously motivate us as an adult-child to seek out an unhealthy partner in an attempt to heal our parents' troubled relationship via our own life.

The unconscious drive behind this illusion is to rewrite the script of our childhood. Thus, our childhood vulnerability often results in a state of reactive adulthood. Only by superconsciously interrupting the negative unconscious states can we establish liberated, authentic self-empowerment.

The Miracle-Making State

As most of this book points out, we are composed of two distinctly different selves, a mortal self that requires miracles and a divine self that creates them. In spite of the confusion that's stirred by the illusion of our mortal identity, accessing our miracle making self is really quite simple.

It's not about doing; it's about being. It's about having the consciousness to know who we truly are.

There is a Divine "I am" within us living side by side with a mortal "I am." What is "I am"? It is having the conscious ability to recognize and know the totality of our true divine nature. Due to *its* willpower, our mortal "I am" appears to have miraculous powers. Mortal willpower can only generate force, and force cannot create miracles; it can only create a need for them. Only by emanating from our Divine "I am" can we access the natural power to create miracles. Miracles are extraordinary events that are the result of the channeling of our own divine power.

Through the knowledge of the Divine "I am," we can achieve the very greatest of possibilities. Being aware of the eternal soul that we are and choosing to consciously channel our highest intentions through that Divine Source will almost always result in miracles.

Most of us have spent far too much of our lives in states of fear, helplessness, and failure. We've been programmed to identify with self solely from the perspective of the mortal "I am." Nothing could be further from the truth than the illusion of the mortal "I am," but it's a myth that has profoundly influenced our broader cultural reality.

We've come to accept the flawed self as our sole self. Whenever we're in desperate need of a miracle, we're inclined to reach above and beyond to those powers greater than we. But there is no power greater than that of our Divine self. I sense that the reason we struggle with the acceptance of our God-self is because of where we think from, rather than what we think about.

In order to overcome doubts about our God-selfhood we must first strive to think from our superconscious God-mind. That's the only place where we'll find enough forgiveness to make room for the consideration of our Godliness. If we think about the prospect of our God-selfhood from our human mind, we'll never get past the self-judgment and guilt.

It is only by embracing our dual nature with unconditional self-love that we can gain access to the miracle making miracle being that we are.

There is so much more to us than we know. We are truly Divine. Each and every one of us is a maker of miracles.

An Exercise to Attain the State of Pure Presence

Take a moment. Stop what you're doing. Tune your attention to each breath. Inhale slowly and smoothly. Exhale fully. Listen to the syncopations of the act of breathing. Draw your attention deep into to your life-generating rhythms. Continue breathing with your complete concentration focused on each breath. Before long, you'll find you are fully present in the field of NOW.

Each breath is timeless. Within each breath there exists an endless lifetime. The timeless space that is created within every breath creates an infinite space for our undivided presence. The undivided presence that results from the power of NOW is a reflection of ultimate power.

A Final Thought on the Presence of Love

We are the fading shadow. We are the eternal light . . .
We are the ephemeral illusion. We are the imperishable truth . . .
We are the forgotten promise. We are the undying love . . .

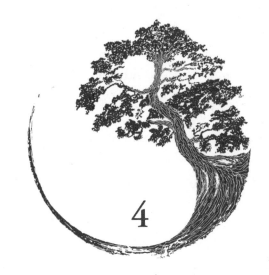

Dis-ease/Disease

Superconscious healing is based on the axiom that most ill health is caused by an absence of ease. Even the cellular, mechanical, and genetic aspects of our physical afflictions are quite often rooted in a chronically dis-eased state of mind. Even though there may be many underlying or secondary causes to an illness, the energy generated by stressors triggers the symptomatic expression of the most chronic maladies.

An Absence of Ease

When I was just beginning my work thirty-seven years ago, I estimated that no more than one in ten of my patients' visits were rooted in stress. Today, it is more like nine out of ten. I shudder to think of the growing number of annual doctor visits either directly or indirectly related to stress. Experts now believe that more of us suffer from stress than ever before contributing to a dramatic rise in conditions such as heart disease, asthma, irritable bowel syndrome, Alzheimer's, Parkinson's disease, multiple sclerosis, and rheumatoid arthritis, to name a few.

Stress is one of the most frequently used words today, but it's a word that is typically used in a meaningless or nonspecific way. In today's world it's almost impossible to go through a day that isn't affected by some sort of stress. What does that really mean? What is stress? Why have we become so dis-eased by it?

On an average day, each human is bombarded with more than one hundred thousand words worth of information. We are deluged with more information than we can keep up with or mentally process. Consider the constant flow of updates most of us contend with: We begin the day with some form of news, check our phones for text messages, check our email, and systematically determine which are most important. At work, we're faced with a load of things to be accomplished, problems to be thought through, issues to be discussed, and maybe some personal issues to sort out around the water cooler. When we get home, there are domestic concerns to be heard and processed. We live every day inundated with information overload. Some of it is relevant; some of it is not. The totality of all this information leaves us feeling overwhelmed.

This tension and strain have us locked us into a perpetual state of fight or flight, and unfortunately, it's emblematic of a cognitive burnout that's severely depleting our brains and bodies. The vanishing ease and flow of our mental states are giving way to a multitude of cognitive and emotional dysfunctions. Our body, mind, and spirit are suffering mightily from our multitasking overload and our addiction to social media. We've created a world of distraction and disorientation that's wrapped up in overwhelming information and tied with a bow of bad news.

Behavioral experts recently discovered that those of us who are insistent on tuning in to negative news are significantly more anxious and depressed then those who don't tune in. Negative news has been found to generate symptoms of anxiety, depression, and even PTSD. Studies have revealed that bad-news junkies tend to spend more time thinking about their worries and have a more difficult time controlling their emotional states. This, in part, is due to the fact that we are more naturally inclined to focus on negative news because our nervous systems are wired for hyper-vigilance, which is our protection against threats to our survival. In this maniacal age of information overload, much of what we're unconsciously downloading is dark and deeply negative. It has never been so important to consciously edit and filter what we allow ourselves to take in.

The mind is engaged in a constant dialogue with the body. Our state of mind exerts a powerful influence over our state of wellness, which makes dis-ease and disease inalterably linked.

In this age of devices and social media addiction, it seems as though we're busier than we've ever been before. Studies reveal that we're really not, but due to the fact that we are connected twenty-four hours a day, seven days a week, we're inclined to feel busier. We are never without our devices, and that, coupled with all other exterior influences, means we are losing our precious connection to NOW and the sacred ease that accompanies it.

Stress

Our disconnection from NOW and the resulting preoccupation with the depressing past and the anxiety-provoking future is the root cause of our disease. The single word that best describes this is *stress*.

The famed endocrinologist Janos Hugo Bruno "Hans" Selye conducted extensive research on the biology of the stress response or what he referred to as the general adaptation syndrome (GAS).[1] Selye, who coined the word *stress*, was the first person to correlate general adaptation with the development of pathological states from chronic uneasiness (dis-ease). He was the first to correlate stress with the hypothalamic-pituitary-adrenal axis (HPA). That all-important connection demonstrated the glandular wear and tear of stress on an organism. It was largely due to the brilliant work of Selye that the world was made aware of the direct association between stress and disease.

Since Selye's pioneering work, the scientific world has learned much more about the biology of stress, as well as the ramifications of stress-borne illness. The process can be explained quite simply. Stress generally begins in the mind in the form of a perceived threat. From there, signals are sent from the mind to the brain to mobilize for fight or flight. Powerful, action-based "super" hormones, including adrenaline, are then secreted. I refer to them as super because they provide the body with a temporary explosion of supercharged energy that enables it to run faster, jump higher, and feel stronger when confronted by a threat. We have heard the remarkable stories of soldiers in the heat of battle who, despite suffering incapacitating wounds, heroically come to the aid of their fellow soldiers. I've often written and spoken about a truly incredible story of a fifteen-year-old boy from the Midwest who miraculously managed to lift a car off of his grandfather. The two were repairing the boy's vehicle when it suddenly slid off the blocks it was jacked up on. It landed squarely on top of the grandfather. In a burst of superhuman strength, the boy power lifted the car up and off of his grandfather, saving his life!

Whenever we encounter stressful situations, the brain's hypothalamus produces chemicals that activate our pineal gland, amygdala, and sensory cortex. The first stage of adrenal reaction to stress is called the alarm phase. Resistance and recovery follow it. Immediately after the body goes into alarm, the adrenal glands flood the body with adrenaline and cortisol, which mobilize the body for fight or flight.

During the alarm phase of stress, adrenaline and cortisol increase the heart rate to prepare the body for a sudden burst of energy to engage in either fight or flight. Next, the peripheral blood vessels in the hands, feet, and skin constrict so that the vital internal organs can receive more blood. The spleen contracts and blood clotting increases in order to offset any potential of excessive bleeding as we fight or flee, the liver releases glycogen to boost energy, and sweat production is increased to lower the rising body temperature. Breathing speeds up, and respiratory passageways expand to facilitate greater oxygen intake, which allows the body to eliminate excess carbon dioxide, a waste product that needs to be removed from the body.

During the resistance phase, enzymes and saliva are decreased, efficient digestion is replaced with emergency digestion, which drops the blood pH levels to an acidic range, and the liver's stored sugar provides energy on demand.

Obviously, stress represents a powerful shift in chemistry. It changes the body from an efficiency state of being to an emergency state in milliseconds. We must not forget that all this powerful chemistry is triggered by states of the mind. While stress states and stress chemistry can save our lives in a short-term necessity, they tend to do serious damage to us in the long term.

Experts tell us that human stress chemistry should be used during 15 percent of our total lifetime. They further believe that anything more than that will only result in exceedingly degenerative wear and tear of the body and mind. Unfortunately, we've managed to de-evolve to the point where most of us are engaging our stress chemistry continuously. Unfortunately, we've learned to thrive on stress without recognition of the perpetual damage we are doing to our whole being.

The Energy of Dis-ease

One of the most important factors in any system of healing is establishing a causal root. That simply means that the patient can't be effectively treated for a given health condition unless, and until, the practitioner discovers where the imbalance originated, where the symptoms are rooted. If the core of the problem is not determined, then the practitioner is doing nothing more than applying a bandage.

We know that stress triggers emotional tension, which causes dis-ease and ultimately disease. This is a sequence of events evolving from energy to manifest as matter. It is our tendency to see life solely from a matter-based perspective; thus, our current Newtonian understanding of medicine is, for the most part, based on our knowledge of cells, tissues, organs, and organisms. Moreover, here in the West, when it comes to establishing the causal root of disease, the prospect of energy remains curiously absent.

Everything, including you and me, is composed of energy. Before we can begin healing with energy, a diagnosis must take place. When energetically diagnosing disease, there are only two possibilities. Disease energy can either be excess or deficiency. The goal, of course, is to ultimately reach a state of balance.

The state of excess represents inflammation. The state of deficiency is degeneration. Diseases such as rheumatoid arthritis, fibromyalgia, and Graves' disease (hyperthyroid) are inflammatory conditions and are therefore generally considered to be diseases of excess. Osteoporosis, Addison's disease (acute adrenal gland exhaustion), and chronic fatigue syndrome exemplify diseases of deficiency.

This is another indication that the Universe is governed by unwritten laws of duality. No thing and no state is ever exclusively based in excess or deficiency, as energy is fluid and forever in flux between two polarities. Things may predominately or constitutionally reflect excess or deficiency, but they are forever blending into one another, back and forth in an unending flow that demonstrates their Universal inseparability. There is an old saying that pertains here. "The darkest of night comes just before the dawn."

Maintaining the principle that everything is energy and energy is a constant state of flux, diseases of excess are always moving in the direction of deficiency and diseases of deficiency are always moving in the direction of excess. The worst cold or flu goes from being extremely symptomatic to stopping because it runs its course. It's like a balloon that expands with each breath, as it simultaneously becomes one breath closer to popping and being empty. We're inclined to believe that opposites are unrelated. We don't understand that there's a mutual compatibility between opposition, and we further don't understand that due to the fact that everything is energy, opposites are therefore not static but fluid.

Like ocean tides rising and falling, each state is in the active process of creating the opposite. Disease is destined for a cycle of wellness, and wellness is destined for a cycle of disease. This is why the practice of disease prevention, a balance and harmony between the polarities, is vitally important.

Dis-eased Mind = Diseased Body

It's the physical realm's inclination to view whole systems as separate entities. Nowhere is this more apparent than with our not-so-holistic perception of mind and body. We separate and compartmentalize the two, but in the world of energy, all is one. The multiverse is but one unified field that is composed of mutually compatible opposites. Understanding that concept allows us to understand and appreciate that there is no separation between mind and body. The natural progression of that thought is that whatever the mind experiences, the body also experiences simultaneously.

Neurologically, there is a biofeedback loop activated within the mind and body circuitry that communicates via the body's bio-energetic grid. This grid represents the unification of our psychological and anatomical energies, giving birth to what is called our psychosoma, the mind and body as a functional unit.

Matter affects energy just as energy affects matter. There is no difference between the two. In the same way, there is no difference between ease and dis-ease. As is true with yin and yang, one force is forever pouring itself into the opposite power where it is then returned to its source. Understanding this interrelationship between ease and dis-ease represents the most important of all fundamental wisdoms that can help us to overcome disease.

The dis-ease that gives birth to disease reveals an incessant subliminal dialogue between mind and body that constantly crosses the bridge between formlessness and form. As that happens, stress becomes emotion that downloads to the subconscious, which ultimately affects the cellular level of the body.

Every one of us is carrying emotionally imbalanced energy that's producing a type of subterranean dis-ease in multiple patterns. These play a role in the underlying cause and origin of illness. It is where dis-ease and ease converge. Ancient classical Chinese medicine clearly grasped the connection between the energy of dis-ease and the matter of disease. Those practitioners believed the energy of anger is stored in the liver. The energy of joy is stored in the heart. The energy of anxiety is stored in the spleen. The energy of sadness is stored in the lungs. The energy of fear is stored in the kidneys. Their wisdom teaches us about the interrelationship between subtle vibrations produced by emotions and how those frequencies positively and negatively affect the physical body. There's much we can learn from those ancient concepts that pertain to the orderliness of disorder.

They understood how repressed or overexpressed anger can disturb liver function, about how repression or overexpression of joy can disturb the balance of the heart, about how repression or overexpression of anxiety can disturb the balance of the spleen, about how repression or overexpression of sadness can disturb the balance of the lungs, and about how repression or overexpression of fear can disturb the balance of the kidneys. The natural result of balance between the energetic and material is healing.

Energy that is repressed becomes inflammatory. Energy that is overexpressed becomes degenerative. In order to overcome the disharmony created by dis-ease, we must make whole the interrelationship between dis-ease and ease as it exists in the mind and body. It's important to decipher the dialogue between ease and dis-ease and mind and body that is generated. That dialogue streams throughout our bio-field, which is the spherical field surrounding our physical body. It is the medium for virtually all dialogue between the mind and body.

Autoimmune Disease

Setting the tone for virtually everything in the mind, body, and spirit, humans have two immune systems: efficiency and emergency. We also have two nervous systems: parasympathetic (ease) and sympathetic (dis-ease). When we are at ease, virtually every system in our body is more efficient. When we are dis-eased, all of the body's systems shift into an emergency mode and are significantly less efficient. When such an imbalance persists, the result is often the onset of autoimmune diseases.

Autoimmune diseases occur when an inefficient immune system mistakenly attacks its own vital tissues, organs, and glands. The human immune system is composed of a powerful army of natural killer cells, T and B cell lymphocytes, interferon molecules, spleen tissue, and specialized antibodies that are designed to protect us against invading micro-organisms like viruses, bacteria, protozoa, and fungi. But serious problems can occur, as I experienced, when a chronically stressed, overtaxed nervous system pushes too hard on an already burnèd out immune system. This, in a nutshell, is how the door to autoimmune disease is opened.

It's commonly accepted that there are over one hundred autoimmune diseases including: Addison's disease, celiac disease, Crohn's disease, dermatitis, endometriosis, fibromyalgia, giant cell arteritis, Graves' disease, Hashimoto's thyroiditis, herpes, nephropathy, juvenile type 1 diabetes, lupus, Lyme disease, Meniere's, multiple sclerosis, PANDAS, peripheral neuropathy, psoriasis, Raynaud's, restless leg, rheumatoid arthritis, sarcoidosis, scleroderma, Sjogren's, and vitiligo.

The common factor among autoimmune diseases is that the body turns against itself. The immune system actually attacks the body. Western allopathic medicine generally turns to immunosuppressive drugs to treat autoimmune diseases. These drugs suppress immunity in an attempt to ramp down the body's confused attack on itself. The problem here, of course, is that by suppressing the entire immune system, you run the risk of rendering the body vulnerable to assaults from other potential attackers such as bacteria, viruses, and even cancer. In essence, an immunosuppressive medicine that might assist with rheumatoid arthritis might also increase the risk of contracting other health impairments. One thing is certain: autoimmune diseases ravage the human body, and the result is chronic and acute states of inflammation. Stress triggers the expression of autoimmune diseases and autoimmune diseases trigger inflammation.

Inflammation

The word *inflammation* has two different meanings. Acute inflammation refers to the body's reparative reaction to injury, and chronic inflammation refers to the body's symptomatic reaction to a foreign substance. In both cases, the body's immune system sends white blood cells to the exposed area and increases blood flow to the tissue, which results in redness and warmth. It can also refer to a buildup of inflammatory compounds called eicosanoids. These can be the cause of chronic disease.

Eicosanoids are super-hormone-like cell mediators that are derived from essential fatty acids that perform vital functions and exert extremely powerful inflammatory and anti-inflammatory effects on the human body. There are three major categories of eicosanoids: neutral, inflammatory, and anti-inflammatory. As is the case with actual hormones, these hormone-like molecules are constructed from the raw materials of fatty acids. There are six essential fatty acids, three of which produce both good and bad eicosanoids. The arachidonic fatty acid is the principal agent from which inflammatory, or bad, eicosanoids are constructed. Alpha linolenic fatty acid represents the raw material from which anti-inflammatory, or good, eicosanoids are produced. The neutral eicosanoid category is derived from the fat linoleic acid.

Chronic inflammation is much more than just an achy joint. The number one killer, heart disease, takes the lives of nearly one in four Americans each year.[2] Cancer, the number two killer, claims about six hundred thousand lives annually, according to the American Cancer Society.[3] Both heart disease and cancer are inflammatory diseases. According to the National Center for Biotechnology Information (NCBI), chronic inflammatory diseases are the most significant cause of death in the world.[4]

Fats come from foods. The food-produced fats stimulate the body's manufacturing of neutral, bad (inflammatory), and good (anti-inflammatory) eicosanoids hormones. In my practice, I have directly linked inflammatory disease with an inflammatory diet!

Foods like red meat, egg yolks, dairy products, and peanuts are high in inflammatory arachidonic acid, which produces the bad eicosanoids that trigger many potentially life-threatening diseases.

My nutritional suggestion for inflammatory disease is to increase foods like fatty fish, flax seeds, and organic vegetables and low-sugar fruits like berries and apricots.

Foods like poultry, beans, legumes, and whole grains produce a neutral fat called linoleic acid that can be converted into an anti-inflammatory eicosanoid with the nutritional supplementation of any one of three linoleic oils. These oils are evening primrose oil, black currant seed oil, and borage oil.

The actual expression or activation of our disease tendencies can be reversed. Anti-inflammatory nutrition can reverse the inflammatory processes, and that can reverse our disease patterns.

Genes and Nutrigenomics

Each of us has a genome that is established during conception. Many experts believe that this life map represents our destiny. Is this true, and if so, to what extent is it so? It is, indeed, a map of possibility. It contains the sum of our DNA, the molecule that holds all the hereditary information necessary for our ongoing construction as a living organism.

DNA was first identified in 1869 by chemist Friedrich Miescher but was largely considered irrelevant until the 1930s and '40s, when a series of germ experiments began to reveal its hereditary significance. Scientists learned that when viruses infect human cells, they inject their DNA into those cells, producing copies of the virus. Thus, science established that DNA contains detailed information and instructions for viral replication. More to the point, they were learning that DNA carries information from cell to cell via specific genes, profoundly influencing the genetic building process.

DNA is contained within genes, and genes are contained within chromosomes. Chromosomes are composed of thin, string-like structures of nucleic acids and proteins and are found in the nucleus of most living cells. Genes within chromosomes are the master carriers of genetic information from cell to cell. This genetic process has an impact on cellular replenishment, aging, disease, and even death.

The outer membrane of the cell is responsible for transporting oxygen and vital nutrients to all other areas of the cell. This is nature's way of ensuring total cell replenishment. The outer cell grows much faster and larger than the inner cell. Ultimately, the overgrown outer cell membrane is unable to reach and nourish the remaining internal components of the cell and the cell must ultimately divide upon completion of its life cycle. Healthy human cells divide approximately fifty times throughout their lifetime with the help of chromosomes. Chromosomes are vital to this process, as they contain all the information and instructions necessary for cell division. Each time cells divide their chromosomes wear down on the ends. This is how aging manifests at the genetic level.

There is, however, a significant response to the aging process provided by nature. Proteins called telomeres cap the end caps of the chromosome structures. You might think of them as something similar to plastic shoelace caps. These telomere proteins serve as protective support for the chromosomal wear and tear of the cell division process that is associated with aging. Research has proven that the aging process can be slowed down by this telomere protection.

Telomeres produce an enzyme called telomerase. This has been shown to protect and, in some cases, repair chromosomal telomeres. This protein is specifically what provides the body with the ability to lengthen telomeres and reverse the aging process.

Our gene map is unique to us alone. It contains our patterns and probabilities for constitutional makeup, aging, and disease. You've probably heard the outdated thought: if your mom or dad had arthritis, you'll likely have it too. When considering our hereditary prospects for sickness, disease, and aging, it may seem a little intimidating, as our gene maps are quite fixed.

The good, and updated, news is that we now know we can alter the expression of our genes in a fraction of a second! It takes nothing more than positive thoughts! Additionally, genetic nutrition, called nutrigenomics, has exhibited the power to radically alter our genetic expression for the better.[5]

Protective telomerase production has been shown to increase dramatically with antioxidant nutrient intake, exercise, and stress management. Scientists have recently discovered that converting dangerous free radical molecules into protective antioxidants helps change the genetic process for the better. Following a Mediterranean diet or simply consuming more vegetables, fruits, legumes, and whole grains can achieve this. Regular exercise and daily meditation are also extremely beneficial protectors of telomerase production. And there are over twenty-five supplemental nutrients, including vitamins A, C, and E, as well as L-glutathione and NADH, that have demonstrated the ability to increase telomerase, thus extending the telomeres and reversing the aging process at a genetic level.

According to a study of 4,676 nurses, appearing in the December 2014 *British Medical Journal*, the nurses who adhered to the Mediterranean diet had longer telomeres.[6] The research documented that those who followed a diet rich in vegetables, fruits, legumes, and whole grains lengthened their telomeres and lowered their risk of chronic disease and overall mortality.

In 2010, a team of German scientists found that fit, active subjects consistently demonstrated 40 percent greater telomere length when compared to their sedentary counterparts.[7] A number of studies have consistently found that dedicated meditators have on average one-third greater telomere length than non-meditators. All this research indicates that genetic life extension is about positive thoughts and super nutrients and optimal nutrition. The lesson of telomeres is that the miracle of disease prevention and longevity are largely a matter of choice.

We once thought of disease and untimely death as a genetic definitive that appeared in the gene map at the time of conception. But our understandings are changing dramatically. We are discovering that our subconscious mind and our nutrigenomic status have more to say about our longevity than previously thought possible. Where our genes were once believed to impose a major influence over causal disease patterns, scientific research is proving that our minds are a key factor in our physical health. There is mounting evidence of the role of the mind in disease and healing, which is leading to a greater acceptance of mind–body medicine.[8]

We are no longer solely the genetic victims of our heredity because now we understand the mind/body connection is real. Ultimately, disease is caused by dis-ease, and superconsciousness is one of the most powerful antidotes for disease.

The Deepest Roots of Dis-ease

The roots of dis-ease can be traced deep within the innermost recesses of the subconscious mind. In fact, their reach may just extend beyond the fathomless depths of time.

I heard a story from a colleague about a patient of his, a woman who'd been suffering from acute migraine headaches. For many years, she sought all forms of Western medical help but to no avail. She tried everything within reason to overcome the crippling headaches and was so frustrated that she was willing to try virtually anything. As a last resort, she decided to work with a woman who was a practitioner of regression therapy. The woman hypnotized patients with the intention of subconsciously erasing their psychosomatic maladies.

During their first session together, while under hypnosis, the woman with the headaches vividly recalled what she recognized as one of her past lifetimes as a bar maid in the Wild West. She saw herself getting caught in the middle of a dispute between two drunken cowboys. Under hypnosis, she recalled that one of the cowboys recklessly drew and fired his gun, accidentally hitting her in the head with a stray bullet that ultimately killed her. In the millisecond just before she died, she reported experiencing a crushing headache the instant the bullet exploded in her brain. She also recalled carrying her migraine headaches into ensuing lifetimes and into this present lifetime. While she was under, the hypnotherapist urged her to release the trauma and reminded her that this event had occurred long ago and was no longer a part of her reality. It worked! The incapacitating headaches were gone at long last.

Based on the diseases and healings I've observed over the years, I recommend past-life regression as a tool to better understand our whole self. Because of the past-life experiences of my patients, I feel certain that the way a person lives and dies in a previous life can strongly influence the patterns of dis-ease they experience during the present lifetime. This is due to what I call *soul imprinting*. The soul represents the immortal self. Imprinting refers to those most indelible events that a soul experiences during a given lifetime. Experiencing inerasable events during a lifetime, such as dying a tragic death, enduring a sudden shocking accident, reuniting with an eternal lover, and even reaching enlightenment can and does exert an enduring imprint on one's soul. The stamp of such an imprinting power strongly influences the subconscious mind and directly influences the current patterns of ease and dis-ease.

Dis-ease germinates at the soul level. It spreads its seeds and roots itself within the timeless, innermost recesses of the subconscious mind, ultimately suffusing itself in the physical body. Like healing, disease is a whole-istic process that reflects a deep entwining between the body, mind, spirit, and soul. Disease is a reflection of our deepest thoughts, dreams, feelings, and expectations. It resides within the recesses of our conscious, unconscious, subconscious, and superconscious mind.

The Subconscious Power of Expectancy

About twenty years ago, a gentleman came see me complaining that simply thinking about spicy food created an instant outbreak of an intense inflammatory skin rash over his entire body. At that time, I'd never heard of such a thing and wasn't particularly inclined to believe him. We talked for a while, and I further questioned him on the matter. At that point I was just trying to flush out his credibility. Nonetheless, I figured it would be easy enough to put his assertion to the test, and after fifteen or twenty minutes of cross-examination, I requested that he substantiate his claim right before my eyes.

The man agreed, and as he sat there before me, I could sense him shifting his attention away from our conversation. His eyes closed, and he appeared to be focusing his concentration more within himself. He explained to me that he was imagining himself eating some food that was doused with hot, spicy cayenne pepper.

In no more than two to three minutes, I clearly saw his perspiration increase. Then, an inflammatory red rash blanketed his entire body in a matter of seconds. I could hardly believe my eyes! He had clearly demonstrated to me that his subconscious mind had generated a power that altered his biochemistry! As much as I had studied and read about it, this was the first time that I'd personally witnessed the reality-altering potential of the subconscious mind.

This moment was a profound life changer for me. *If our minds have such power*, I remember thinking, *just how much do our thoughts commonly influence our manifestation of disease?*

I eventually put him on a bland diet, taught him to meditate, and guided him to visualize that he was rolling in a snowbank as a method of reversing the inflammatory effect.

Of course, since that time, much has changed. Back then, determinism was believed to be purely genetic. Science now knows that the fate of our cells is also determined by the conditions of our environment, both our physical and mental environments, which are ultimately one. The brain translates the mind's images. The images we picture in our mind create a specific correlative chemistry in the body. Love and gratitude give birth to wellness. Resistance and resentment are harbingers of disease. The status of our cells is continuously shaped and reshaped by the perceptions of our mind.

The reality-making power of the mind has been scientifically validated by decades of research on the placebo and the nocebo effect. Placebo effect has proven that we will tend to produce a beneficial effect by believing that we can. Nocebo effect suggests that we'll tend to produce a negative effect by merely expecting it.

It's becoming clearer that, through expectancy, we create what we anticipate and expect as the end result. Dr. Walter Cannon studied tribal death from voodoo curses and found that a number of otherwise perfectly healthy subjects, who died shortly after being cursed, had in fact died only because of their expectation to succumb to the curse.[9]

Similarly, Helen Mayberg's work discovered that regardless of whether a patient received prescribed antidepressants or placebos, the same areas of the subject's brain were activated, validating the material power of belief and expectancy.[10]

This phenomenon has always been central to my work. I will forever encourage my patients to charge up their positive beliefs and expectations to boost their miracle healing potential. It's what superconsciousness is all about. This healing expectancy can be reinforced with hypnosis. Hypnosis can help us to remain positive and stress free. It's about maintaining such a strong belief in extraordinary outcomes that the extraordinary outcomes are, in reality, created by the power of the belief.

Eighteen miracle stories that defy medical logic are the subject of three documentaries I've produced or coproduced. These events happened, and each miracle maker openly shared their story with the world. In every one of these cases, the patient engaged the subconscious power of expectancy.

One such story had to do with a fifty-year-old male patient who had been diagnosed with end-stage prostate cancer. I immediately put him on an anti-inflammatory diet and instructed him to avoid dairy, red meat, nuts, fermented foods, corn, egg yolks, and wheat products. I also supplemented his program with the herb pawpaw, ellagic acid, and black cumin seed oil caps.

It took only five months for him to reverse his cancer. While I'm certain the diet and supplementation were very important, I am convinced that his relationship with his wife and their relationship with God had more to do with his miracle than anything. Both he and his wife exhibited a superconscious strength and positivity that was uplifting even to me whenever I was in their presence. They were a force of positive expectancy that absolutely willed him to beat his cancer!

It's very important to recognize that our subconscious mind never turns off. Therefore, we have a choice to maintain experiential programming that is rooted in negative expectancy or to position our thoughts and come from a place of belief and expectancy where we are always creating a more dynamic result.

Exercise to Create Positive Expectancy

We have been taught to anticipate the negative aspects of life so that we can avoid them. That may be an important part of the material world survival manual, but it limits our ability to create and manifest from the positive core energy of the Universal mind. There is an ancient exercise that has been practiced by Tibetan luminaries for thousands of years. Throughout the centuries, it's been used to greatly empower a heightened sense of positive expectancy and magically make miracles happen. Read through the following prompts. Then close your eyes and keep them closed until you've completed the step-by-step exercise. Some people prefer to use their smartphone or other device to record and play back the prompts.

In your mind's eye clearly see your desired miracle.

Envision the black void of space all around you.

Visualize a shimmering metallic star off in the distance.

Project your expected miracle through your third eye (between your eyebrows) outward to the distant radiant star so that the star can absorb it.

Once the star has absorbed your expected miracle, take in and absorb the energized miracle within your mind through your third eye.

Envision the star exploding three successive times in your mind, as you then draw the star down into your heart for three more successive explosions.

Finally, draw the star out your third eye and back out again to the Universal black void.

Perform this manifest exercise twice each day, three times per week to power up your miracle expectancy—and just watch what happens!

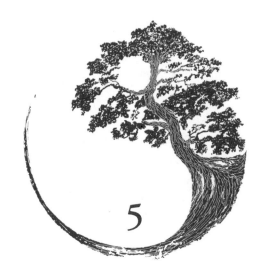

The State of Ease

Miracle making begins with superconscious living. Superconscious living demands that we expand our awareness to understand that our life was created on purpose so we might live *in* purpose. Purpose is synonymous with ease, and ease is the antidote for dis-ease.

Ancient Taoist sages believed that at the moment of conception, every infinitesimal detail of our true nature was etched into our hearts. This sacred inscription is said to reveal our source, the truth about who we truly are, as well as our life's purpose. The sages further believed that as we evolve in consciousness, it was incumbent upon us to recognize and know these revelations that are hidden deep within the inner sanctum of our being. It is our responsibility to determine the purpose and flow of our life and the ease with which it can be obtained.

Purpose

The word *purpose* generates great energy, as it reflects the power of meaningfulness. It speaks to just how plugged in we are at the level of heart, soul, and mind. Living in purpose suggests that we are consciously dedicated to attaining precisely that which is destined for us. It's about living in a manner that clearly demonstrates we're not here simply to take on life's material challenges. Purpose is far more powerful than that. It's actually a state of mind that becomes energized by the higher frequencies of heart, soul, and mind. By living in purpose, we activate the flow of a powerful vibration.

The power of living in purpose often competes with conditions born from pleasure and pain. In the grand scheme, these two conditions have much to say about our mastery of living in purpose. Pleasure can inspire us forward, just as it can hold us back. Pain can also inspire us forward, just as it can hold us back. Human nature has a penchant for the paradoxical, especially when it comes to the duality of pleasure and pain. Pain makes us feel. In a world that has all but forgotten how to feel, feeling anything can feel good.

Beyond that, there is a powerful release of energy that comes from the pain that forces us to feel. Many of us are subconsciously attracted to circumstances and people we know will present us with the most painful karmic challenges. Such a perilous attraction can ultimately force us to get in touch with the kind of intense emotion that will empower us to move beyond them. This serves us by making us formidable in the end, or as the German philosopher Friedrich Nietzsche eloquently stated, "That which does not kill us makes us stronger."

It's very important that we tune in to the internal subterfuge of both our pleasure and our pain. The subconscious attractions to such adversarial relationships may even reveal a hint of seduction. We often become addicted to that which hurts us most, simply because it pushes us beyond the entrapment of our own repression. Each of us is the primary obstacle that gets in the way of reaching our higher purpose. It is not the perpetrator that we've selected as our karmic villain, as much as we'd like to place the blame on them. It we who are the obstacles in our own way.

Ultimately it comes back to the question of ease versus dis-ease. If ease is resisted, some form of forceful disharmony, or dis-ease, will always be the natural result. This is no different than a drowning man who insists on struggling against the tide. All the energy in the Universe is moving in one direction, but because its elusive ways evade our sometimes senseless senses, we disregard it. We relegate ourselves to the resistance of dis-ease.

The ease associated with living in purpose is nothing short of transformational. It has to be. The fulfillment of each and every higher purpose fuels and sustains the very life force of the entire Universe. Our innate Universal nature has installed an infinite supply of fail-safes to make sure that everything moves forward and the most crucial things always are accomplished. Anything that resists the ease of living in purpose will be forced to contend with those Universal fail-safes. Therefore, anyone who fails to live in purpose fails to generate ease and will be forced to contend with the repercussion of dis-ease.

It's crucial that we release anything that's holding us back from living in purpose, as it will have an effect on the entire Universe. By living in purpose, we are each contributing to the wholeness and flow of the Universe. The purposeful path can be very narrow, as we set ourselves up with the lessons taught by pain. Dysfunctional relationships, jobs, friends, enemies, disabling emotions, negative thoughts, overwhelming conditions, and deeply troubling circumstances can be painfully obstructive.

Perhaps the most difficult part of this process might be distinguishing the difference between letting go and not hanging on anymore. Letting go has the distinct benefit of gravity. Just release your grip, open up your hand, and let nature take its course. Letting go isn't an action; it's a nonaction. Once we make our peace with the concept of releasing their grasp, flow will follow faith.

The act of not hanging on anymore is an action. It's an action that does not have the benefit of gravity and therefore must generate all its own volition and power. Not hanging on represents the action of disposing of or casting away something that is a detriment. That is much more difficult than opening one's hand and letting gravity rule.

When we talk about releasing all that's holding us back, we're all too often referring to long-term interpersonal relationships that have, over the course of time, become intolerable. In far too many cases, despite all the burdensome pain and suffering caused by these relationships, there's a subconscious desire to hold on to them. This perceived need to hold on "for dear life" is really not related to living. In fact, it's often more of an emotional death grip that can drain all the precious life right out of us.

Throughout this "holding on" process, there is often a protracted deliberation where we obsessively weigh and justify the means against the ends. Internal conversations may go something like this: *Should I or shouldn't I stop hanging on? When and how should I stop, if in fact I can?*

If we are hanging from a cliff and let go, we fall. No longer hanging on to something conceptually implies we are taking a dive. With that in mind, one of the most compelling questions of all is, Do we have a protective safety net in place for the hard fall we may be about to take? Throughout this painful process of not holding on, we tend to forget that we've already suffered the most damaging plunge of all: allowing ourselves to fall from the highest grace of our own Divine purpose. That is the most damaging freefall a human soul can take. It's essential to recognize that whatever we stop holding on to is holding us back from our living in the natural flow of our own divine purpose.

In the final analysis, the only real decision we have to make is just how long we're willing to suffer. It may require several attempts to release that which is holding us back. But one way or another, we will let go of those things that restrain us. Every action and reaction ultimately aligns with the way of purpose.

Flow

Flow and resistance are the central themes of most ancient healing philosophies. Chinese, Ayurvedic, and ancient Egyptian medicine all believed dis-ease to be the natural consequence of blocked energy, which is resistance. According to these primordial systems of medicine, impeded blood flow, blocked lymph filtration, and repressed emotions are considered the most common harbingers of the energetic dis-ease that can, and probably will, devolve into physical illness. Ease, though, is synonymous with flow, healing, wholeness, and wellness. But the dis-ease that results from resistance is and always has been common and ever present in life.

Imagine that you awaken to a new day, effervescent, filled with enthusiasm, and very much at ease. As you begin your morning, you are suddenly embroiled in a bitter dispute. You do everything in your power to rationally resolve the conflict and return your life to a state of ease, but your adversary is vehemently resistant.

It doesn't take much opposition to derail the flow. It might be something as immaterial as an irritating text, an annoying email, or a road-rage-aholic riding your bumper on the drive to work. These are just a few examples of some of the common forces of resistance that can rise up against us on any given day. None of us are strangers to the dis-ease of resistance, which robs a lot of balanced energy from us, whether we recognize it or not.

Resistance and flow represent the very basis of energy. Resistance is the tangible effect of unnatural force. It reflects the detrimental defiance of the predestined forward motion of universal energy. Flow is the affirmative movement of energy as it is the exemplar of natural power. Flow is the Universal torrent that animates the unceasing tides of life. Flow escorts every scintilla of Universal energy directly to its singular place of destiny. Resistance will be broken and shattered by the sheer force of its own illicit nature.

Though resistance and flow are diametric opposites, they have one distinct thing in common. They are both highly charged manifestations of energy. While there's no question that resistance is indeed a negative force, it is, unquestionably, mighty. That's exactly what makes its energy so potentially valuable. Imagine being able to convert the thrust of such force into positive flow!

Our material education has programmed us to believe that our only recourse for dealing with a resistant force is either to fight force with force or to ignore it. But in the world of energy, there is another option. It's called transmutation. With transmutation, you don't fight it or hide from an opposing force, you convert it.

Einstein taught us that energy can neither be created nor destroyed, but it can be transmuted. This means that every form of energy can be transformed into another energetic form. So, the next time you are confronted with the adversarial forces of resistance, you might consider the option of transmuting that potent force into the positive power of flow.

For centuries, practitioners of the martial arts of jujitsu, aikido, and judo have mastered the transmuting of their attacker's resistant force by reconstituting it in such a way as to work against the foe. Energy mastery such as this represents a reality that's radically different from what we're accustomed to in the Western world. When it comes to the transmutation of energy, we have much to learn from the ancient east.

Chi Gong is an ancient Eastern form of energy mastery capable of instilling great transmutational powers in its practitioners. Many years ago, I viewed a presentation where a Chi Gong master implored a dozen or so would-be attackers to aggressively advance toward him. By vigorously waving his hands toward the ground, he transmitted an incredible bolt of energy that was so powerful that it knocked every one of the attackers down, even though they were some thirty feet away. Without physically touching them, the master transmuted the energy of the attacker's force in a way that redirected it against them. They were driven to the ground in a matter of seconds. There they lay frozen in place, unable to move until the master once again shifted the energy in a way that allowed them to rise off the ground. It was truly remarkable to watch.

Chi Gong provides us with important clues regarding the development of our transmutational potential. It teaches us that by developing the domain of great mental powers, or what is called the *yinias* or *yi con-sciousness*, through visualization and precision focus, we can gain access into our limitless superconscious mind. There energy can best be recon-stituted. The extraordinary powers of Chi Gong are created from within the mind. It is through the mind-body grid that massive energy fields made up of photonic emissions are generated. To date, there are more than 1,600 research papers that demonstrate this. Graphic mental visualization, unwavering concentration, and powerful intent enable the Chi Gong mind to access realms of transmutation. The power of dynamic thoughts such as these enables us to invoke transformative changes back and forth, between energy and matter.

The ancient Chi Gong pioneers believed there to be two minds: the mind of emotion and the mind of intent. The mind of emotion is sometimes referred to as the place of a thousand streams. The mind of intent is said to represent the one great stream. You get a clear idea from these descriptive references that the mind of intent is a domain where powerful, superior focus is believed to reside. Focus of course can be distracted by emotion. Thus, by disciplining the mind of emotion and by focusing our mind of intent, we put ourselves in a strong position to master Chi Gong or, more specifically, to transmute the force of resistance into the power of flow.

The Chi Gong form that I implement to transmute resistance into flow is called Wenchiech'u. It's simple yet powerful. It is all about visualizing vigorous spiral motions in the mind's eye and then transmitting the spiral of energy to a subject. The ancient masters taught that spirals visualized in the mind were representative of extremely powerful agents of energy transmutation that could be projected nonlocally to any distance. Counter-clockwise spirals are seen as yang, or energy stimulating. Clockwise spirals are believed to be yin, or destimulating. Any person, place, or thing that is energy deficient can be stimulated and thus balanced by counterclockwise spiral motions. Any energy that is excessive can be destimulated by clock-wise spirals.

Let's imagine that some form of adversarial aggression has confronted you. Where your aggressor's energy is clearly excessive, your transmutation process is going to want to reduce the energetic charge of their wrath with clockwise spiral projections. It's important to keep in mind that the greater the negative force of their resistance, the greater their conversion to positive flow. The bigger the fish, the harder the fight, but the more mouths it will feed.

Creating Ease by Releasing Dis-ease

The ancients understood that there can be no healing ease until the resistance that blocks flow is released. Much of our dis-ease is rooted in obstructed negative emotion. When we experience physical or mental pain caused by another and hold tight to bitterness and resentment that results from the experience, we only serve to prolong the karma and intensify our dis-ease.

The deeper inner workings of refusing to release and the struggle that accompanies release probably has a lot to do with the human desire to control. We don't have much mortal control in this life. Basically, there is no control over birth, the aging process, or death. Throughout the entirety of our life experience, we surrender a great deal of control to other aspects of life. Because of this, most of us suffer from at least some modicum of control addiction.

The opposite of releasing, of course, is holding on to. Holding on to represents control and releasing represents surrendering control. We may be addressing the fact that we are holding on to something bad, but it still represents control. Oddly enough, the fact that it is bad can elicit a strange "feel good" effect.

When someone hurts us, the aggression is likely to ignite a fire of anger within us. Anytime such a spark touches off a volatile flame, it is generally going to arouse our ire. That type of emotional disdain tends to get under our skin! Holding on to something so negative can, and often does, result in what I call the refuse-to-lose mentality. In turn, that stirs up an obsessive, compulsive, and possibly addictive response. Letting go of anything so emotionally compelling can be very difficult. The more we try to separate ourselves from it, the deeper it is inclined to burrow within our psyche. Bitterness and resentment have a way of igniting fires that burn out of control.

Many patients I've encountered have intensely suffered in body, mind, and spirit, due to the dis-ease caused by bitterness and resentment they've harbored for long periods of time. Prior to working together on a deeper level, most remain convinced that the solution to all that ails them simply comes in some form of a tiny, colored pill or another shot of alcohol. These addictive methods that we use to numb pain seem to be part of our cultural story. We believe all solutions are contained in the material world. Thus, we remain virtually without a solution regarding those potentially far reaching dilemmas that are rooted at a deeper soul level.

When we hold on to bitterness and resentment from the past, it generates negative frequencies within us. Those frequencies have the power to sabotage virtually every aspect of our lives, including our most precious relationships. When one carries hostility from something that happened in their past into a new liaison, the new relationship is often subverted by the old.

Someone may well have caused you to be hurt, but that was then. It's you who has assigned it a place in your ever unfolding now. It's not about them anymore. It's about your insistence to keep it alive by holding on to it. When that happens, you are not the only one suffering. Those you love most are also suffering because they don't have the opportunity to enjoy a more whole version of you. At that point, your grip on bitterness and resentment is hurting you and those you love far more than the original hurt that was perpetrated on you. The solution is to release it.

As we strive to move beyond the hurt and pain of our past, we must remind ourselves that we've lived many lives and faced a myriad of challenges in those lives. Those lifetimes have given us the opportunity to expand our consciousness and move ever closer to our destiny of pure enlightenment. Sometimes reaching that destination can be difficult, especially when it requires the karmic challenge or prompting of affliction or suffering. Growth and development can be painful.

This is what the superconsciousness way of miracles is all about. It presents a significant challenge to our spiritual acumen. It shifts our perception and reasoning to a higher plane, and transcendently uplifts our awareness far beyond a mundane level. It's our choice as to when we're ready to accept and acknowledge that all paths lead forward toward the destiny of our enlightenment.

Peering through the lens of superconsciousness reminds us that the pain and suffering that incite bitterness and resentment are by design. They are catalysts intended to challenge us to at last turn our gaze to the light of our liberation.

As is the case for all our great tests, it's ultimately a matter of free will. We make the selection between evolution and devolution.

Will we choose to transmit our being-ness through the channel of personal or Universal consciousness? The only reason we've been presented with the gift of consciousness is to evolve the very gift of consciousness that we are. We are pure energy that has come into a state of existence in order to infinitely expand and to ultimately blend with the mind of God. Bitterness and resentment are but illusions of a fictitious reality that is, and forever was, destined to fade into abeyance. But their karmic presence in our lives has a purpose. The pain and confusion that arise from bitterness and resentment can ultimately draw us to enlightenment. Due to the basic need to release and let go of the pain, suffering, and the confusion that they produce, we are ultimately drawn to the light.

Most of us are mistakenly inclined to associate the prospect of enlightenment only with those few, rare, exceptional souls, like the Dalai Lama and Mother Teresa. The mere mortal nature of the physical self makes it difficult to be associated with such an exalted possibility. However, enlightenment is the ultimate destination of every soul. Each and every one of us is on a journey of a thousand steps: two forward, one backward. It is a voyage for both saints and sinners, all of whom have come solely for the purpose of transforming beyond the mortal limitations of karmic confinement.

As eternal souls, we come to this polarized world of sacred tension only to release our dis-ease and to be drawn to the ease of the eternal light. The ultimate goal is to attain enlightenment, and in the end, we will know and understand that every single step has been necessary.

Paying Down the Karmic Debt of Dis-ease

Spiritually speaking, dis-ease is a reflection of karmic debt, a debt that can only be paid down with the currency of enlightenment. The greater the karmic liability, the more spiritually impoverishing the dis-ease. The more spiritually impoverishing our dis-ease is, the more one needs to invest in the wealth management of superconsciousness.

Only by the actions and reactions of transgressions does the soul create karma. When confronted with the most important, challenging choices, poor decisions activate the power of our karmic gravity.

Bad karma is a corrective reaction to imbalance, and it is powered by suffering. It's the transgression that perpetuates the suffering and the suffering that creates the dis-ease. The incessant festering of the dis-ease burrows deep within us to reveal the name and face of the karma we've created. Dis-ease is born of bad karma.

It could be no other way, for the Universe is forever consciously observing and correcting itself. A wrong decision on our part and the suffering begins. It must begin because the Universe, which includes each of us, is in a perpetual state of self-corrective counterbalancing.

The Universe is pure consciousness that is eternally seeking flow. We are part of a macrocosm that is in an eternal state of expansion. The corrective forces that represent the way of things summarily devour any energy that resists the flow of the natural expansion of the Universe.

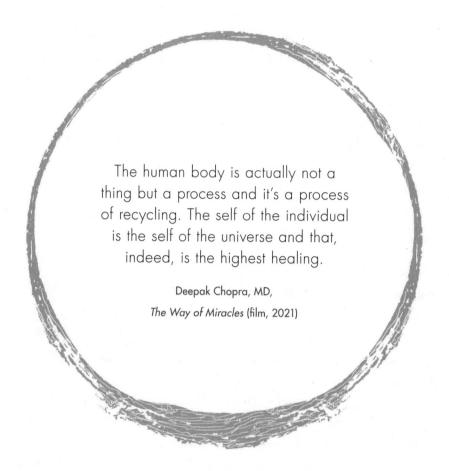

The human body is actually not a
thing but a process and it's a process
of recycling. The self of the individual
is the self of the universe and that,
indeed, is the highest healing.

Deepak Chopra, MD,
The Way of Miracles (film, 2021)

When it comes to change, the Universe represents both cause and effect. It is forever changing us. But because we are the Universe, we also have the power to change all that changes us. There is a natural interchangeability between the Universal microcosm we are and the Universal macrocosm to which we are inextricably bound. As the Universe rights itself, we right ourselves. Many of us are going deeper within to quell our suffering from dis-ease by paying down our karmic debt. This may be why we see our world currently experiencing a transformational renaissance.

Deeper, more personal forms of spirituality are replacing well-established institutions, such as organized religions. Increasingly overwhelmed with karmic suffering, many souls are searching for more from self, each other, and the innermost depths of source.

Mindfulness has become a personal destination for many. People are searching for deeper meaning within themselves and in their relationships. It's as if we are awakening from a nightmare where everything extrinsic has all but lost its once fundamental meaning. Nationalism, religion, love, marriage, and family have all suffered cultural deathblows. That, in turn, has pried open a pathway to explore our connection to source.

Everywhere you look, you see people struggling in the throes of a turbulent transition. A mass reordering of our lives is taking place. The change is within us. After all, we are the Universe that's dictating the changes we are being forced to contend with.

It is due to our own self-manufactured bad karma that we've created the need for the very transformational challenge that now stands before us. The only way around it is through it. The only way we can truly create ease is by paying down the karmic debt of our dis-ease with the currency of pure light.

The Every-thing-ness of No-thing-ness

Surprisingly, our present ethos, with its absence of belief in miracles, represents the perfect void from which to build a bridge to a new ethos. The phenomenon of no-thing-ness that naturally arises from an ethos absent of miracles reveals a great contradiction, perhaps one of the greatest paradoxes of all. Confronted with no-thing-ness, the only possibility that remains is that the door to every-thing-ness can open.

We've all experienced more than our fair share of emptiness, such as when we pray from the deepest depths of our soul for a miracle, but try as we might to force it to manifest, our miracle is nowhere to be found. That's because it's not supposed to be.

The reason it's not supposed to be has to do with the source from where the would-be miracle is derived. Generally, when we feel powerless, we're inclined to reach out beyond the boundaries of self. We look for a helping hand or a boost up from any form of "other." And when we pray, we tend to pray outward and upward to that "other," which we assume to be greater than we are, for deliverance. We've all been codependent victims of an ethos of "other." "Other" represents everything around and above self, but in this instance, it seems that there is no "other." It appears as though all "other," even our creator, has abandoned us.

No-thing-ness implies a time of great desperation when we pray to God unceasingly, without an answer. It's as if no one's out there. We might even feel as though God has chosen to ignore our desperate pleas for help and our family, friends, neighbors, spirit guides, and guardian angels have turned their backs on us as well.

Such desperation brings to mind the Old Testament book of Job. Though "blameless" and "upright," God took everything away from Job: his home, his seven thousand sheep, his three thousand camels, his five hundred yoke of oxen, his five hundred female donkeys, his servants, his friends, and even his seven sons and three daughters. God wanted to test the depth of his faith. Job eventually asked God why he was condemned to suffer so undeservingly, but he was provided with no answer. He was simply left with no support, no answers, nothing more than his deserted self. There were no miracles anywhere in sight. If there was going to be a miracle of any kind, it was going to have to come from him.

In the end, Job discovered that he was responsible for changing his perception of suffering. It was through his faith alone that he was able to experience the everything that comes from nothing. And so it is with us. It isn't about being fulfilled by all that is around us. It's about being filled full from that which is within us.

When the entire world around us, and all the heavens above us, turn away, it's the Universe's way of telling us to turn inward and turn to our miracle creator self. No-thing-ness allows us to clear the way for the ultimate miracle that naturally arises from the abolition of codependency, the cultivation of personal autonomy, and the birthing of self-sovereignty.

Miracles of grace that come from without last a lifetime. Miracles of greatness that come from within last an eternity.

Ease from Detachment

There is an ancient Chinese saying that suggests that the best way to clear muddy water is to leave it alone. This is the way of ease. When you have a conflict or problem that's part of a spiritual lesson, do you have the strength to simply leave it alone? We're programmed in this culture to exercise the willpower of our ego and to assert ourselves over our problems with force.

The detachment that produces ease demands that we channel our problem-solving through faith and surrender with total confidence in the way of things. By elevating our consciousness, we put ourselves in position to allow for the Universe to solve problems from within a higher dimension.

During your life, how many problems have you experienced that were exacerbated by an overbearing nature? Here in the West, we pray for outcomes in which we expect God to intervene. By so doing, we're demonstrating a kind of faith that requires surrender and a degree of surrender that requires detachment. Is it not also true that there is a way for the Universe to exercise its gravity over all things including our problems? If we can exercise faith in God, then why do we struggle to hand our faith over to God's Universe?

Detachment doesn't exclude us; rather, it consorts with the higher part of us where the will of our ego merely engages the basest part of self. If you have the power to detach in such a way as to allow the Universe to produce your result, do you then have the strength to detach from all ensuing conditions? It's one thing to hand over your problems to the Universe; it's another thing to detach from the result. The Universe and its way of things has the perfect reason why not to provide us with our ego's desired result from time to time. Can we put as much enthusiasm into unconditional joy, faith, trust, and acceptance of the result of our problem when the solution does not satisfy the desires of our ego?

By detaching, it appears that we leave ourselves suspended from the gravity and grounding of our own still point. In fact, by detaching from one reference point, we ironically become attached to another. By detaching from our lower energy, we attach to our higher energy, and by detaching from our mortal self, we attach to our immortal source. Finally, by detaching from the concept of a separate self, we attach to interconnectedness or our universal self.

Detachment brings us swiftly and directly to every frequency associated with superconscious ease. By cultivating such a frequency, we instill our whole being with the potential for miracles. Those patients with whom I've worked, even the ones with terminal illness and dire conditions, who were able to detach themselves from results and maintain an elevated vibration, consistently experienced the most miraculous outcomes. Detachment results in superconsciousness, and superconsciousness produces the ease that results in transformational healing.

The Internal Source of Ease

Not unlike a stone that's dropped into a pool of water, the ripples move from the inside out. The healing energy that ultimately extends outward to our cells, tissues, and organs is initiated deep within the core of our innermost being. The flow moves from the internal to the external. Thus, healing must begin by establishing a rudimentary vibration of ease within the mind, spirit, heart, and soul.

It is our proclivity to identify with disease from what I call the pain point. For example, if someone has a headache, the practitioner is inclined to focus their attention on the patient's head; if the patient has a stomach ache, the practitioner's attention will most likely be drawn to the patient's stomach. We tend to go to wherever the symptoms express themselves.

In point of fact, not unlike the rippling water example, the problem is almost always initiated at a deeper internal level, so the headache might have begun with an emotional repression of anger or stressful frustration. The stomachache likely had origins at an emotional or deep-thought level. With this in mind, we find that not only disease but also healing takes on a whole new meaning.

By directing our healing attention to the internal, we are much more likely to get to the root of the dis-ease. In addition, there is a greater likelihood of teaching one to prevent disease. This all becomes much more instinctual at the energetic level as energy tends to manifest as matter.

The source of all ease is internal. For us to become miracle-making superconscious healers, we must learn to direct our wellness focus on the energetic origins of the dis-ease at the most subtle energetic and ethereal levels of our being. Our diagnostic systems, our therapeutic solutions, and our way of life must become more adroit on the subtle vibrational plane. This is the way of ease.

By evolving from doctoring the body to healing the whole being, we revolutionize our understanding of ease. To live our lives at this subtle vibrational level represents a quantum leap where our miracles will, at last, manifest without self-restriction.

We belong to the Universe, we are the Universe, and we contain a Universe within. It is our internal Universe that reflects our Divine Source, and it is from our Divine Source that we perform the greatest of miracles with ease.

Transmutation Exercise

Get started by simply turning on your mind's eye and focusing in on an image of your adversary. This can be performed nonlocally. Regardless of whether they are standing next to you, in the car behind you, or a thousand miles away, you can transmute their energy from the dis-ease of resistance to the ease of flow by superimposing clockwise spirals of energy over their image in your mind. This process requires only that you draw the dis-ease out. The Universe will naturally replace it with ease. It only takes a minute and a half to two minutes to deliver and set the charge. One single two-minute spiral projection can last up to one week, but it may take up to one full day to take effect. Feel free to perform additional boosters; it's safe to do that but not really necessary.

Remember, you are always the clock, facing outward. Therefore, clockwise will always spin to your right, and counterclockwise will always spin to your left. Counterclockwise spirals can be projected successfully in the same manner to those who are weak and lack energy. By combining graphic visualization, strong intent, and superior focus, you will be afforded access into the yinias, or the domain of great mental powers. Here, you can alter energy in ways that serve the greater good.

One very important point to note is that the power of belief is a prerequisite for transmuting energy. We have easily adapted to constantly evolving technology, yet we resist adapting to the ancient physics of energy. Few of us understand how the car remote can transmit a flash of unseen energy that can unlock their car door or even start the engine from a hundred feet away, yet no one ever questions it. Nor could most of us explain how live images of people, places, and things can magically appear from the distant corners of the earth and outer reaches of space via an internet video call, but magically, they appear in the comfort of our own home. Without understanding how or why it works, we accept it and know that it will be available when we need or want it.

In order for our practice of Chi Gong to effectively empower us with the ability to transmute energy from negative to positive, we have to develop the willingness to believe and a consciousness of confidence.

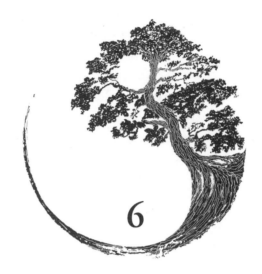

The Transpersonal Shift

The word *transpersonal* is used in various schools of philosophy and psychology and is defined as "the areas of consciousness that are beyond the limits of personal identity and ego." It's representative of the state of awareness that exceeds the material realm to the point that it is unifies with the consciousness of the universe.

Most of us exist in the realm of personal consciousness, but in order to access the power to make miracles, a transition is required to a more thorough, deeper transpersonal awareness that flows with that of the Universe.

Access to superconscious power is proportionate to the vibrational frequency in which we reside. Maintaining the transpersonal state causes our vibrations to elevate to the very highest frequency. Meditation, prayer, singing, dancing, immersing ourselves in nature are all ways to elevate and maintain our frequency. The higher our vibration is, the greater our access to boundless potentials. When we self-identify in a comprehensive, unified way, we become one with the infinite and thus gain access to its power.

It can be difficult to step away from the material world and recognize we are infinitely powerful. We've been indoctrinated to accept that we are a narrowly defined, isolated, incapable, and powerless being. We've been instilled with the doctrine of "can't," and we have believed it without question. Subsequently, the acceptance and appreciation of personal power remains deficient and the potential to make miracles remains unrealized.

It is time to expand our cognizance beyond limited material perceptions of reality. That can be achieved through a shift to transpersonal identity, which requires expanding the recognition of realities beyond the material world.

There is much more that is real than what we see before us.

The theory of transpersonal superconsciousness aligns with realism that stretches far beyond the third-dimensional five senses. This theory proposes that there's much more to life than our material senses can perceive. Just because we can't perceive it doesn't mean it doesn't exist. There are as many dimensions of reality as there are states of consciousness to access them. It's like a hall of mirrors.

With the awareness of transpersonal superconsciousness, the whole game changes. Reality takes on a quantum perspective that represents a new paradigm, where every mind has open access to unlimited possibilities in the realms of the infinite.

Dimensional Shifting

Transpersonal denotes states of consciousness beyond the worldly, mundane perspective. It speaks to a different reality, a quantum reality where energy and matter are synonymous. It's a paradigm that is based on quantum mechanics rather than classical mechanics. This is where time and space are considered illusions and the quantum baseline aligns perfectly with superconsciousness.

When we think of miracles, we tend to get stuck in the debate as to whether they do or don't exist. But the more valuable question is: Are we ready to recognize that miracles require the three realms of higher dimensional transpersonal consciousness?

The Three Realms of Higher Dimensions

- Astral realm, which is soul emotion

- Mental realm, which is abstract thought

- Causal realm, which is spiritual thought

You might be asking, "How do we get there?" There are five primary brain wave states that are vehicles to access these higher dimensions.

The Five Brain Wave States (Vehicles to Higher Dimensions)

- Beta, 14 to 30 Hz, alert/hypervigilant (blocked from higher realms)

- Alpha, 9 to 13 Hz, relaxed (accesses astral realm)

- Theta, 4 to 8 Hz, deeply relaxed/loss of body awareness (accesses mental realm)

- Delta, below 4 Hz, meditation and trance (accesses causal realm)

- Gamma, 30 Hz, bursts of transformative awareness (expands in causal realm)

Quantum Consciousness

The quantum mind conditions of theta, delta, and gamma are domains of consciousness that we're much more familiar with than we may realize. We experience these brain wave states more often when we're children because childhood is a time when creative invention is encouraged. Imagination blossoms into nondimensional reality.

The last time you gazed out a window, lost in the beauty of a field or forest that stretched across the horizon, were you taken to a trancelike state? Did it feel like you were actually there in the midst of the vision? You were! Your soul essentially traveled to astral, mental, and causal planes.

By disengaging the tether to material reality, we begin to experience the transcendence to the serene pathways of our consciousness. When we look out a window and feel consciousness projecting over the tree-tops in the distance, the astral light body is, in fact, actually flying over those trees. Some might say that is nothing more than imagination. But consider a premise with roots in Hindu belief that fosters the concept that in addition to our physical body, we are also made up of four light bodies: an etheric body (the ether energy field around the physical body), a mental body (the energy field generated by the mind), an astral body (the energy field generated by emotion), and a ketheric body (the causal body energy field linked to the creator). Light bodies are not bound or restricted by time and space. They are the vehicles that transport us through our superconscious evolution and from personal consciousness to universal consciousness.

We haven't been taught to observe nonphysical realities even though they exist. Access is impossible unless one dwells within these quantum states, fully conscious, and with clear intent. Most of us are just random visitors who accidentally drop in and drop out of these realities in an unconscious manner. The realms of higher dimensions are extremely fertile places of superconscious power that can be cultivated by deep meditation and trance, and once they're harnessed, they can open the door to unlimited miracle-making potential.

Trance

Every miracle is born of thought, and every thought is born of mind. Every human mind is capable of producing a myriad of varied states, some of which are substantially more powerful than others. The mind possesses the ability to initiate and ultimately realize complexities that range from the magical to the mystical, if it is properly developed and nurtured.

Trance states have long been thought of as the mind's birthplace of the improbable, if not the impossible. Our ancestors used rituals to reach a trance state and did so with the intention of reaching realms of the extraordinary. Primitive human beings discovered that trance states greatly assisted with their spiritual experience and miraculous healings. Some ancient cultures mastered techniques or trance exercises as a way to reveal the portals of power and healing.

Accessing Portals to the Infinite

Practicing the soul-traveling, portal-opening exercises at the end of this chapter increases the power of your quantum, superconscious, manifesting potential. They should be practiced as often as possible, at least once per day, to advance your awareness of these unseen dimensions and the capabilities that belong to them. Frequent practice establishes faster, easier access to these realms, and eventually you'll skip the soul-traveling-portal exercise all together because you'll be synced to the energy of your miracle potential in an instant.

Energy is ubiquitous. It embodies the Universal reservoir of infinite potential. In order for energy to manifest as a desired outcome, it must be directed. Human intention is one of the most, if not the most, powerful catalysts to cultivate energy. With it comes a broad range of motives and possibilities that can be generally categorized as good intention, which is cultivated by superconsciousness, or ill intention, which is generated by ego consciousness.

Quantum Manifest

The best way to engage in the process of making miracles is through manifesting. *Manifesting* simply means "to make something happen." Each of us has the power to make miracles happen, but to do so, we must first be willing to challenge our views that limit our perceptions of reality.

One of the most substantial falsehoods of earthly perceptions is that reality represents a fixed, collective absolute. That is to say, we assume that we're all viewing the same movie of life from a similar vantage point and arriving at uniform conclusions about what we're observing. It's an assumed concept that is hazardous to our soul's development.

The fact is that in the quantum universe, each separate observer uniquely influences reality. That power of the observer calls the very perception of reality into question. That is called the observer effect, and it exposes that phenomena are actually altered by acts of observation.

An example is the double-slit experiment, a noted physics experiment that demonstrated that light and matter have the ability to display characteristics of both of the classically defined waves and particles of light and matter but that are determined by the observer. We assume that a table and chair we're looking at are part of a fixed reality. But by just looking at them, observing them, you're actually altering their properties and thus you are influencing reality.

In October of 2017, researchers from the Institute of Optics in Palaiseau, France, discovered that by bouncing photons off of satellites, an observer could influence whether the photons behave like particles or waves.[1] Those changes were made solely through observation.

Cocreating Reality

Reality is not fixed, collective, or absolute. It is a fluid, relative absolute.

If a tree falls in the forest and nobody observes it, it eludes quantum reality. Why? Because quantum reality requires the presence of an observer, and in the case of the falling tree, it's only a reality to those observers who actually witness it. It's through our presence as an observer that we become authenticators of reality. And it is through this power to determine reality that we become cocreators.

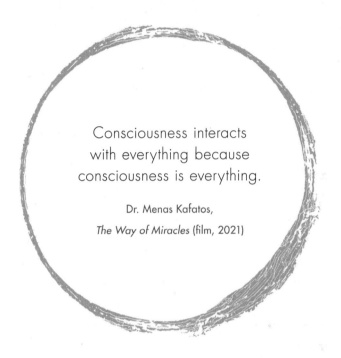

Consciousness interacts
with everything because
consciousness is everything.

Dr. Menas Kafatos,
The Way of Miracles (film, 2021)

According to quantum mechanics, reality isn't based in a set of governing laws and standards that operate outside the field of our conscious experience. It is the uniqueness of our conscious perception that perpetually sets and resets the reality we observe. That makes each of us, individually, the observer-creator of our own unique and ever-changing reality.

If you and I are walking down the street and a blue car drives by us, we automatically assume that we both saw the same shade of blue. The truth is, there are over a million shades of color perceived by the average human eye, and each of us tends to see varied shades of every color. Some of us have what are called vortex eye cones, which perceive over 100 million shades of color! The probabilities are high that you and I are likely seeing a different shade of blue car. The same holds true for what we hear. Let's assume that the driver of that same blue car beeps the horn. Are we both hearing the same sound? With over 425,000 audible tones, we are probably hearing audible tones that are at least slightly varied.

It's the relativity factor that places reality squarely in the observer's field of perception. The key is that the observer is not restricted to a passive position. Recognizing that every observer is experiencing their own unique reality empowers them to cocreate. The observer can decide to cut the tree down or deny that it ever fell. Belief is the empowering variable.

In a world that needs to define and limit reality, what you get is what you see. In the realm of quantum reality, what you see is what you get. The realm of quantum reality is the powerful foundation of and to manifestation.

If we agree to live with self-imposed limitations and cultural indoctrination, we will struggle with the concept that we have access to unlimited powers to manifest. Self-doubt, personally perceived limitations, including our mortality, and the fear of being judged by others prevent us from advancing to quantum manifestation. But a simple willingness to believe is all that this transformation process requires.

It might seem to be a bit of a catch-22: If you don't believe in your ability to generate, or at least access, unlimited power, you won't make miracles. If you don't make miracles, you won't believe in your unlimited power.

Quantum reality manifestation is an action-based proposition that becomes energized by belief. The only way to break the cycles of self-limitation is to embrace unconditional belief and to engage in constant action with deliberate expectancy. That unconditional belief and constant expectancy generate energy that alters matter and changes fate.

Human life experience may begin with vulnerability, but the greatness of our story can only be written as it unfolds. We are the authors of our destiny and the miracle making greatness of our story is entirely up to us, the authors.

It's not a matter of reaching miracle-making greatness through performance. True greatness has nothing to do with material achievements. It's not about having a productive day, week, month, or year. We're conditioned to believe we only deserve the label of greatness because we accomplished some achievement in the material world.

What we tend to ignore is that we are immortal souls. Recognizing and accepting that as fact gives us the ability to embody true greatness. By consciously emanating from the soul, we inhabit the state of our greatness. Living in a permanent state of greatness is realizing and believing in our immortality and allowing that knowledge to flow from the source. It's about making the decision to transform the perception of our identity from a random ego to an eternally conscious soul.

Shifting the perception of reality from randomness to consciousness and from codependent to cocreator is what quantum reality manifest allows us to do.

Greatness is not reserved exclusively for the Mother Teresas, award-winning scientists, and superstar athletes of the world. They are not better because they achieved something most don't or can't. The bedrock of greatness is ultimately a matter of relative reality.

Each and every one of us has experienced challenges in our lives. The outcome of adverse events was, whether we knew it or not, largely dependent on our personal perception of reality. Did we choose a reality to overcome or to succumb?

Manifesting represents a supreme action state. It has the power to alter fate. If we are engaged in the quantum process, we are no longer just entertaining a vision, we are transmuting the energy of vision into material form!

Manifesting is an act of creation that evolves from intent to event. For example, you might hold a vision that depicts you writing a bestselling novel. In the early stage of the vision, you're working at pure thought level, but before long you have a novel in hand and are looking for a publisher.

Power generated by such a vision can provide the necessary inspiration to convert thought energy into material reality.

Einstein's theory of relativity serves as a constant reminder that energy and matter are interconvertible or capable of being exchanged on an equal basis. Energy and matter are transferable. Every thought we think is matter that holds unique and varied energetic potential. Thoughts about putting on your shoes and socks are simply not going to generate the same energy as thoughts about making passionate love. That's because thoughts originate in different domains of our mind. There are four primary domains of mind: conscious, unconscious, subconscious, and superconscious, and each of these has their own unique tendencies.

The conscious mind is adept at initiating and reinforcing goals.

The superconsciousness represents our most exceptional mind as it represents a merger with divine awareness.

You can activate the power of your superconscious mind via meditation (alpha brain wave) or trance (delta brain wave) states. Cultivating the next level of this higher mind power requires going beyond deep relaxation and merging our consciousness with God-consciousness.

The final step entails empowering your quantum manifest intention. While there has been a recent surge of interest in subconsciously driven accomplishment, most of us attempt to reach goals simply by engaging our power of concentration. But if we consciously connect our human mind with divine mind, we significantly bolster the power of our manifest potential.

It's about rising up and expanding our power far above and way beyond the mundane. In virtually every aspect of life, there is always a higher level to attain to. When we infuse our personal perception of reality with belief in infinite expectancy, we awaken from mediocrity and walk in the radiant light of our true miracle-making greatness.

The Transpersonal Vacuum

Vacuum is defined as a space totally devoid of matter. Consciousness is not a material substance, but does it exist in a void? Noted theoretical physicist and philosopher John Archibald Wheeler is widely recognized for his research on the space-time continuum and for coining the term *black hole.* Wheeler proposed that every single bit of matter in the universe contained consciousness. The consciousness in all matter was obtained from the proto-conscious field of awareness that surrounds the universe, which means the Universe is actually a living being that has a conscious field of its own and we are an integral part of its totality.

Transpersonal denotes the areas of consciousness beyond the limits of identity or ego. The vacuum is the void. Together they indicate that our consciousness fills the void. Reaching the power of the proto-consciousness is about being aware that you are in the zone when you are actually there!

Once we comprehend the fact that we're an intrinsic element of the proto-conscious field, we can access the power to manifest from within the quantum vacuum, simply by elevating the vibration of the mind. Nothing will raise our vibration more than simply becoming aware of our higher awareness.

The quantum vacuum has been defined as a zero-point field that contains no physical particles. According to quantum mechanics, it's anything but empty. It contains fleeting electromagnetic waves and particles that pop in and out of existence. It represents our mind's open access to virtually everything. It opens a door to limitlessness.

There are two ways for us to enter the quantum vacuum. One way is to cultivate a more refined consciousness in our day-to-day life or, as previously stated, to become more conscious of our higher consciousness. We can accomplish this by becoming the meditation and prayer. It's less about creating a momentary meditative state and more about cultivating a permanent meditative domain that is fed by positive thought and reinforced with expectancy of good.

The other way is to frequent the deeper states of consciousness such as alpha, delta, theta, and gamma. Trance states have been proven to expand consciousness and enhance mental powers. Practicing the Trance State Exercise and the Portal Exercise at the end of this chapter are helpful with both methods of familiarizing oneself with the quantum vacuum and can help access all of the limitless power of the proto-conscious field.

Transpersonal Sustainability

We are each a reflection of many different selves. At any given moment, on any given day, we might be expressing any one of a number of our varied dispositions and temperaments. We are reactionaries to exterior influences. One moment we might appear fragile and powerless and the next moment vibrant and determined, but rarely do our responses pertain to the present moment.

Reactive or reflexive actions are generally associated with a stimulus of past trauma because we're neurologically wired to react to adverse memories or conditions that might trigger them. Sometimes our efforts to shape an elevated reality are deterred because of reactions that have nothing to do with the present moment.

Our nerves and muscles actually hold energy associated with memories that can be unconsciously triggered by association. A place, a fragrance, or a painful anniversary date can put our psyche in a state of negative unconscious reaction. When we recognize an association from a past event that influences our response, it's time to overcome its manipulative sway over negative, unconscious reactions. If we prevail in the release of those past traumatic triggers, it's easier to cultivate a more elevated personal reality through conscious, positive pro-action.

To be fully engaged in our abilities to make miracles, we need to constantly check in on and actively renew our commitment to consciousness. While sustained transpersonal awareness holds the key to maintaining a state of positive pro-action, it also prevents negative unconscious reaction. This is how we shape reality.

Maintaining sustained transpersonal awareness means that we concentrate our cognizance, sharpen our mindfulness, and deepen our superconsciousness on a moment-by-moment basis. It's like an ongoing, waking meditation that enables us to mentally scan and rebalance our total state of self. Imagine the clarity that comes at the end of a twenty-minute meditation. Envision the exact same effect without closing your eyes or withdrawing to a quiet place. The most important part of this process is to continually rescan and re-examine ourselves throughout the day, every day, always mindful of our state of consciousness. Unfortunately, there is no way around it: life is distracting. We need to be able to recognize that we have fallen back into old habits and make a correction immediately. The cultivation of sustained transpersonal awareness is the single most empowering process that any human being can engage. It allows one to clearly see patterns of entrapment in negative, reactive thought and reminds us that it's always a matter of choice as to whether we shift to a more positive proactive mindset.

Sustained transpersonal awareness clearly reveals the sharp edges that distinguish the boundaries of self-contrast. The more our consciousness is exercised, the more precise its exacting vision becomes and the more inclined we are to see our self and our life through the honest lens of the soul. Basically, via sustained quantum awareness, all flaws and falsehoods regarding the illusionary depiction of self are placed under a spiritual magnifying glass.

When the light of our consciousness is turned on, the lucid moments that result remind us that the soul, not the ego, represents our true, limitless, eternal being-ness. In this state, we are inclined to perceive our awareness of self super-positioned high above and far beyond the mundane. Anytime that light of sustained quantum awareness is turned off, we are prone to slip back into the haze of unconscious, negative reactivity. It's easy to lose our footing by simply failing to sustain the light of consciousness. But it is through this process that we learn that the empowerment of positive, proactive living is a choice—a choice that begins with sustained consciousness.

Requiring nothing more than the activation of deeper mindfulness, we can swiftly rescue ourselves amid any psychological free fall. By prioritizing the engagement of sustained transpersonal awareness, we infuse ourselves with the power of choice. Once awakened by our enlightening consciousness, we are empowered to discern and select positive over negative and action over reaction. It is truly remarkable to observe and to experience.

It's always such a pleasure to see this process in action with my patients. When a patient starts to drift into the swells of emotional distraction, I offer a reminder that they've fallen into the trap of unconscious, negative, reactive thinking. I ask if they want to choose conscious, constructive, proactive thinking and establish the advantages of the positive choices.

Most people immediately shift to the positive with a word prompt: consciousness. It's as though the mere mention of the word *consciousness* has a way of activating a homing device that elicits a spiritually sobering effect from deep within the soul. While the act of re-awakening is indeed important, it's even more important to encourage and inspire ourselves to sustain the process.

Life is very distracting, and we humans tend to lose focus. The power of focus is crucial. Concentrated attention on the development of moment-to-moment higher consciousness wakes us from a type of spiritual slumber. It speaks directly to the purposeful challenges of soulful evolution and spiritual maturity. We didn't come here to remain stagnant. We are here to develop and flourish beyond the consciousness and the being that we were when we arrived.

Even though we didn't arrive with a spiritual identity, we have the opportunity to attain spiritual maturity, if we so choose. One's spiritual identity is shaped by choices—choices accompanied by the karmic challenges of free will. How we build and shape our spiritual identity is entirely up to us as individuals. It's fully dependent on the nature of self-programming. We become who we think we are. We manifest self with the same technique that is used to manifest all things. We construct self from vision and the energy of thought ultimately gives birth to the total form of our being-ness. Spiritual maturity takes the same shape as our evolving, or de-evolving, perception of self. As long as we remain conscientiously dedicated to the power of awareness, doors to wonders and miracles remain open to us.

The Transpersonal Peak Experience

Peak experience, or PE, is described as a euphoric, profoundly fulfilling moment attained through self-transcendence. It's believed by some to be a transpersonal state that is capable of inspiring miracles. Noted psychologist Albert Maslow once described PE as, "Feelings of limitless horizons opening up to the vision, the feeling of being simultaneously more powerful and also more helpless than one ever was before, the feeling of ecstasy and wonder and awe, the loss of placement in time and space with, finally, the conviction that something extremely important and valuable had happened, so that the subject was to some extent transformed and strengthened even in his daily life by such experiences."[2]

A team of Norwegian researchers recently conducted quantitative peak experience studies on a group of world-class performers from the fields of management, sports, and music. They found that during periods of PE, subjects reached opposite states of complete control combined with a complete loss of control. And they occurred simultaneously! The paradox didn't end there. These world-class performers displayed unique brain wave activity that resulted in calmness and happiness, and dynamic wakefulness that often resulted in effortless perfection. The exceptional performers also excelled in tests that reflected a higher moral development, suggesting that they possessed a significantly stronger drive to satisfy the needs of others and not just themselves.[3]

PE research has proven that zones of heightened consciousness, trancelike focus, and positive feelings of Universal unification result in transformational human potential. By consciously deepening our mental states and reformatting our brain to expand thought potential, we enter a pathway that borders the cusp of a very different paradigm—one that crosses over the mundane and ventures into the quantum realm.

Everything is energy. Energy vibrates. Along with our heart, the mind and the brain are the vibrational centers of our being. Our brain is composed of 100 billion neurons capable of trillions of synaptic connections. Each connection represents up to one thousand signals per second, resulting in three hundred to three thousand thoughts per minute. Most of us don't realize that we are capable of such vast thought creation. Thought neurons travel up to 250 miles per hour as they transmit thought impulses that result in an endless sea of neurochemicals. Once this synaptic process is completed, physical thought becomes reality, and beyond the neuro-mechanical aspect of thought lies a veritable universe of thought energy.

Thoughts are infinitesimal waves that first manifest at the quantum level. It's at this level that thoughts have been described as rolling and collapsing microbursts of light that generate electromagnetic fields of energy that ultimately vibrate to the point of cognition. This is when the energetic properties of thought are afforded access to the miraculous.

Several years ago my mother hired an arborist to clear some brush and fell some trees from around her Cape Cod home. Everything was going as planned, and then suddenly she heard bloodcurdling screams coming from her backyard. After chopping a large oak tree, the arborist had slipped in such a way that the heavy tree landed directly on his leg, pinning him down and trapping him. He was losing a lot of blood and was immoveable. My mother called for emergency help at once but was gravely concerned about his blood loss. Determined to get him out from under this tree weighing hundreds of pounds so that she could wrap his leg to slow the bleeding, my seventy-five-year-old mother grabbed ahold of that tree and was somehow able to reposition it just enough to be able to access the man's injured leg. Emergency help soon arrived, and the man survived. There's no doubt that that man's life was saved because my determined mother had a very timely peak experience.

From the material perspective, a thought is a thought. In the quantum realm, thought has far greater potential. Thought is representative of energy governed by a very different kind of mechanics. Thoughts that prompt peak experiences are believed to be vibrational microbursts of light. The very word microburst implies the momentary peak and explosion of energy. Does this suggest that the PE can never be more than a purely momentary experience? No. Can we make this wondrous phenomenon last throughout the day? Yes. We have the ability to live in peak experience energy.

Peak Transpersonal Living

We are part of a Universal modulating flow where nothing is static, nothing remains the same, and everything is forever evolving. The nature of our evolution is, at least in part, a matter of volition. Free will partially defines our journey. We can choose to cultivate a higher consciousness that results in peak experiences and we can further evolve in such a way as to extend from peak experiences to peak living.

Peak experiences employ a state of heightened awareness and boundless possibilities, but only in increments of moments. Peak living provides the option to attain such a state with relative permanence.

The questions that loom before us must be reviewed and honestly answered. Are we, as individuals, willing to transform our thinking about who we really are and what we're potentially capable of? Are we ready and do we want to expand our belief in the limitless power of our consciousness, irrespective of what we have been told to believe is possible? And do we need to institute a foundational change of our personal ideology, especially regarding our perception of self?

Answers are found in a very personal and sincere appraisal of who you think you are and who you want to become. This is not as easy as it may sound as it requires releasing the old and welcoming fresh beliefs. Each of us has a dual nature, and it can be a tremendous challenge to free ourselves from the shadow cast by our physical realities and the labels assigned to our physical boundaries. Each of us, including myself, has spent more than enough time in our lives drowning in a sea of iniquity. We have a dark side, but we are composed of an equal part of light. As deep as our darkness runs, so ascends the radiance of our light.

The very microbursts of light that define peak experience come from us! In fact, they are us! We are light, and it's through the light of our superconsciousness that we can make peak living a reality.

Our unseen light body holds the purpose to ascend in consciousness so that we may merge with the creator. The light body is our vehicle for that ascension process. It is also the perfect vehicle for the manifestation of peak living, for it is the very source of light from which sporadic microbursts of peak experience are derived.

We are capable of reinforcing the process of peak living by utilizing the power of expectancy, which ratifies the belief engendered by the positive shifting of personal ethos. The prospect of peak living means that we must maintain conscious priority in order for it to happen.

Thoughts, and the mind from which they come, are directly linked to infinite possibility. Nebulous wanderings of the mind can be trained, and negative thought power can be shifted via positive action. Maintaining peak performance as a part of daily life requires all of that and compels us to reach the state of superconsciousness.

In the superconscious state, time is suspended. That means a peak living experience can be extended far beyond the moment, and by consciously occupying the state of NOW, we have the capability of staying in the *infinite present*.

The current times we're living in are anything but ordinary. The universe, our world, and each and every one of us have been thrust into a radical transformation. The stressful energies we're all currently contending with demand extraordinary spiritual centering. Where prayer was once enough to cultivate a peaceful spirit, incessant prayer is now necessary. Where meditation was once sufficient to cultivate peace of mind, becoming meditative is now essential. Where it was once sufficient for us to spiritually benefit from attaining peak experience, we now have the need to stay in the infinite present so that we might live in peak state. This is all about raising our vibration so that we might overcome the pain, confusion, and stress of our current transformational demands. I've developed a simple but powerful exercise that helps us to stay in the infinite present.

Exercise for Living in the Infinite Present

This exercise can be performed either sitting or standing. First, close your eyes. Begin with your hands by your side. Now, take a deep breath as you slowly raise both hands up to your heart. As you do this, say, "I," quietly to yourself. Imagine that as you raise your hands up toward your heart, you are gathering and consolidating the energy of your authentic eternal self. Next, as you return your hands back down to your sides, release your breath and exhale. Repeat this exercise twice more for a total of three times. This exercise should only be done once daily and is best performed during the daytime.

Among the truly powerful aspects of this exercise is the internal pronunciation of the word *I*. This affirms the true self, whose presence exists eternally in the infinite present.

An Exercise to Reach a Trance State

The trance state enables us access to our higher miracle-making mind. Delta waves, found below 4 Hz, induce a deep relaxed state that allows the body to heal and repair. They are like a slow, steady heartbeat and are generated naturally in the deepest forms of mediation. Delta waves suspend external awareness and permit the freedom to explore superconscious potentials.

For this exercise, search YouTube for music that contains the 3.2 Hz delta waves. Find a piece that is comfortable to you. SleepTube has several 3.2 Hz audio files online.

It's best to utilize this music only when you are able to completely relax. Participation and muscle testing have shown that the best way to experience this is to sit or lie comfortably, close your eyes, and listen for no more than ten minutes. This prepares you for your portal journey.

Portal Exercise

The most direct way to connect to quantum superconsciousness is to soul travel the superhighway of the mind. It's here that human potential can take a quantum leap into a field of infinite possibility. It's a simple three-step process, and once you access the portal, you will be able to feel yourself flying.

This is an exercise in peace and all-knowingness that will strengthen your manifest potential by leaps and bounds each time you engage. If you want to truly experience the power and magic of this state, you must maintain a crystal clear intent and completely let go of all mental clutter, negativity, and confusion. A quick way to let go is to repeat the mantra of *I* for ten minutes.

1. First, breathe deeply and slowly, relax, and allow your uncluttered mind to fly freely for a few minutes.

- Notice the free flow of gentle, cosmic intelligence that easily provides automatic answers to all your deepest questions.

- Simply rest in that state for a few moments as you feel yourself showered with ever-flowing wisdom.

Your theta meditative alignment with the Universal frequency, which is technically 432 Hz, is followed by intention visualization. This will supercharge your manifest power.

2. Immediately following the meditation, take just a few moments to visualize the successful attainment of one important discernible goal.

- Once you are settled in the meditative state of manifestation, it is essential to begin propagating your field of higher intention in your mind. By seeing your attainment completed in your mind's eye, you are initiating and energizing your manifest goal. You will discover that what you are visualizing will soon happen in your day-to-day life.

- Each time you enter this state via your quantum meditation, it's important that you seed another manifest vision, adding to your ever-expanding manifest field of intentions.

3. Finally, take about five minutes for a grounded re-entry.

- Stretch your fingers and toes and gently roll your neck as you reacclimate.

- Acknowledge that you are strengthening your manifest powers by frequenting this process so that whenever you want to perform your healing and/or personal growth miracles, you can more readily access the portal.

Practice this exercise and return to this state of awareness often to gain instant access to the portal door of manifest power. Transcend the ordinary, cultivate greater wisdom, and deepen your knowledge as you explore your quantum potential.

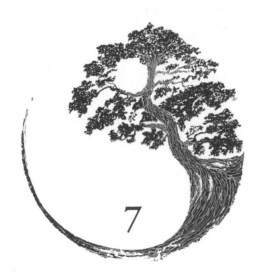

7

Superconscious Healing

The most advanced manifestations of healing are attained through superconscious advancement. There are two superconscious concepts that directly relate to body consciousness. These are embracing wholeness and balancing energy. In these instances, consciousness has two distinctly different perceptions: a heightened state of spiritual awareness and the more generally understood, material form of consciousness, such as health consciousness, dietary consciousness, and body consciousness.

Superconscious Medicine

Energy medicine and nutritional therapy are vital aspects of superconscious healing. Transcendent physical healing can be achieved through conscious systems of energy medicine and nutritional therapy. If it weren't for energy medicine and nutritional therapy, most of my patients would have never experienced the miraculous recoveries that they did.

I created The Whole Health Healing System (MarkMincolla.com) as a contemporized, energy-based, nutritional approach to individualized diagnosis and medicine. It requires precision testing of each subject's organ and glandular strengths and weaknesses, as well as identification of food intolerances. Superconscious nutritional therapies are then designed and implemented for the purpose of supporting patient healing. The nutritional component of superconscious healing begins with food, superconsciousness, and clean eating.

Food Superconsciousness

Hippocrates is credited with the quote: "Let food be thy medicine, and let medicine be thy food." To a degree, he was right. I take it a step further. I used to say that food is medicine, but now I like to say that food is a drug. Drugs can take lives, and drugs can save lives! Therefore, food is a drug. It just depends on the circumstances in which food is used as a drug and its application as a remedy. Superconscious healing is very much centered in the belief that, if properly designed, nutritional therapy can be medicinal, if not outright miracle making. It all starts with consuming a clean diet that is free of chemicals, preservatives, and toxins.

Unfortunately, our world is devolving in an increasingly toxic direction with each passing day. Our bodies have become inundated with artificial chemistry. The more artificial our world becomes, the more synthetic our foods get. The more synthetic our foods are, the more injurious their effect is on our health. Today, much of our food is nutritionally depleted, and some is even toxic. The toxicity of our food supply has become the preeminent destroyer of our health.

The regrettable realities of chemical fertilizing, hybridizing, and growing times that are sped up all act as agents that deplete the food supply of nutrients long before they ever leave the farm. Once they reach the marketplace, our foods, which are our nutrition resource, are assaulted by food manufacturers who proceed to cold store, dry or dehydrate, salt, pickle, sugar, ferment, smoke, freeze, or can to artificially preserve and enrich them. Studies show that such treatment accounts for approximately 80 percent nutrient loss.[1] Even worse than the nutrient depletion of our foods, manufacturers are now poisoning our foods with dangerous toxic chemicals. Among the stockpiles of chemicals added to our foods today are dyes, bleaches, emulsifiers, antioxidants, preservatives, flavor enhancers, buffers, sprays, acidifiers, alkalizers, deodorants, gases, drying agents, curers, fortifiers, hydrolyzers, anti-foaming agents, anti-caking agents, and hydrogenators. There are thousands of cancer-related deaths each year due to food additives.

This is especially disconcerting since recent studies show that the average American consumes approximately 140 to 150 pounds of food additives per year.[2]

Our foods are fatted, sugared, and even genetically modified. Produce is grown with synthetic fertilizers or sprayed with inordinate concentrations of deadly pesticides and its DNA is even altered.

Top all of that off with the way many Americans eat, and there's a disaster in the making. The standard American diet, whose acronym is appropriately SAD, is partially responsible for ill health in all generations. By some estimates, nearly three-quarters of the total calories we Americans consume now comes from highly processed foods.[3] This includes an increasing intake of highly toxic pesticides.

The disturbing facts about the deteriorating state of American food are clearly getting the attention of the whole world, as many of the packaged foods on our grocery shelves are banned in other countries.

Superconscious Nutritional Therapy

Superconscious healing is whole-istic, meaning that it includes body, mind, and spirit, and not surprisingly, it also includes a healing nutrition plan. This ultra-refined process is highly evolved, but it is also highly evolving. As our awareness expands, we are inclined to experience perceptions and attunements that alter and expand our view of reality. One helps the other evolve.

With the advancement of our superconsciousness, we are likely to note significant shifts that accompany our mental, spiritual, and soulful progression. You may find that you develop a greater awareness of the unseen energy of the food. You may actually be able to feel the subtle effects of the foods on your plate, even before it reaches your mouth. That is because the properties of the food are not just present on the physical or chemical level but also exist on the subtlest energetic level.

Superconsciousness elevates our awareness and attunes our vibration in such a way that it makes us more sensitive to energy in general. When we converge with all other forms of energy, who we are is altered, as well as how we are. This is especially true of the influence that food has on our electromagnetic field. Any advancement of consciousness serves to harmonize us with food in an altogether different way.

Most of us don't tune in to the fact that simply hearing the name of a food stimulates energetic reactions within our own energy field. Three decades of energetic food sensitivity testing has repeatedly demonstrated that the mere calling out of a food by name is more than enough to prompt a definitive energetic reaction or response. Everything is energy, and this is especially true of our superconscious relationship with food. This amplified sensitivity renders a distinct advantage to any energy-based nutritional program and has always been the essential difference maker with my miracle-making work. It's at this level that I've been able to consistently generate a medicinal quality for food.

As is true with virtually every aspect of Western living, reality is based on matter alone. Orthodox medicine focuses on the cell; nutrition is centered on nutrients that can heal that cell. Thus, everyone diagnosed with the same given condition is prescribed the same medicine. The whole world is instructed to eat blueberries because they're so nutrient rich that we assume they're good for everybody. This appears to work just fine in the material world, but we need to bring energy into the equation. Einstein made it clear that reality is based on the fact that energy and matter are two parts of one whole. How can we possibly exclude half of reality and be operating at a complete and functional level?

Materially speaking, we all may appear to be pretty much the same on the outside, but energetically, we are all completely separate Universes unto ourselves. This is what separates the superconscious healing nutrition plan from all others. It is energy based and individualized and therefore is not just another one-size-fits-all approach. The exacting aspects of *energy based* and *individualized* combine to empower this as a true "food is medicine" plan.

Superconscious Nutrition 101

Your superconscious nutritional plan begins with setting up a general classification of foods. All foods fall into one of two categories: they are either toxic or they are medicinal. All highly processed junk foods fall squarely into the toxic category.

Toxic Foods

Processed sugars

Fried foods

White flour

White rice

Cakes

(Toxic Foods, continued)

Pies

Cookies

Ice cream

Fast foods

Soft drinks

Juices

Inflammatory foods (red meat, peanuts, dairy, sugar, egg yolks)

Medicinal Foods

USDA Organic, free-range poultry

Wild fish

USDA Organic produce

Herbal teas

Pure low-total dissolved-solids water (water with low levels of potentially toxic residues)

Anti-inflammatory foods (fatty fish, soy, walnuts, pumpkin seeds, flax seeds, organic fruits, and vegetables)

Inflammatory foods are those foods that either contain or produce arachidonic acid, a fatty acid that results in an elevation of what are generally believed to be disease-producing COX-2 eicosanoid hormones. Anti-inflammatory foods are those foods that produce alpha linolenic acid and are commonly believed to produce disease-reversing COX-3 eicosanoid hormones.

The word *inflammation* no longer refers to a simple case of achy muscles or joints. It's no longer singularly associated with injuries or arthritis. We now know that much of our disease is triggered by the chemistry that produces inflammation and is directly linked to the eicosanoid hormone. This does not relate to gender-based hormones. The eicosanoid hormone is believed to be among the most powerful biochemical agents of change in the human body.

There are bad eicosanoids, and there are good eicosanoids. Bad eicosanoids can trigger our body's expression of inflammatory disease, and good eicosanoids can induce a powerful, anti-inflammatory, disease-healing influence. All these stealth eicosanoids, both good and bad, are manufactured from fats, and fats, of course, come from foods. Inflammation is a "bad fat versus good fat" proposition. Bad fats do harm while good fats provide food with a more medicinal power. Junk foods are off the docket, and all inflammatory foods need to be avoided as well, as they put us on the fast track to disease. From a dietary standpoint, we need to learn how we can reverse inflammation. Begin by being aware of the five major dietary influences that drive up our proinflammatory levels.

The Five Major Proinflammatory Foods

1. Red meat

2. Dairy

3. Sugar (high starch)

4. Egg yolks

5. Omega 6–rich nuts and seeds and their oils (such as hemp seeds, sunflower seeds, and peanuts)

Superconscious Nutritional Diagnosis

The primary items to eliminate are junk or processed food and foods that cause inflammation. Food-sensitivity testing allows us to energetically diagnose and record individual responses to foods, as well as test for any potential vital organ and glandular imbalances.

We are composed of energy, and our foods are comprised of energy. Every time we eat, we generate an energetic reaction. Some food sources we consume align in balance with our constitutional, DNA-like energy, and some things we eat create an imbalance. Eating results in one of three things: an inflammatory effect, a balancing effect, or a degenerative effect. That's because with energy, there are only three possible outcomes: excess, balance, or deficiency. Your goals are to embrace your wholeness by balancing your energy.

There are a number of muscle-testing systems that effectively determine the most energetically compatible foods for a given person. I want to share two with you. One allows for self-testing, and the second is called the EMT Surrogate Protocol. EMT means electromagnetic muscle test. This is a relatively simple system that requires three people, one practitioner, one surrogate, and one test subject.

The PPF Self-Test

Let's begin with the personal form of testing. I developed an easy method for a self-testing diagnosis called PPF, Punch Pushing the Fist. This is a pass/fail method for analyzing foods that will help balance your energy.

First, make a tight fist with your nondominant hand (left hand for right-handed people). Place your fist directly in front of your heart, approximately three inches away from your chest. Bend your arm and raise your elbow so that it is level with your fist. Place your dominant hand (right hand if you're right-handed) in front of the nondominant fist. The dominant hand should be farthest from the body. Verbally call out the names of foods such as: apples, beef, chicken, salmon, blueberries, radishes, or whatever food you need to test. As you call out each food, press the dominant hand against the nondominant hand and toward the chest. Repeat the process with each food you want to test.

If there is strong resistance when your dominant hand pushes against your fist, the food is beneficial. If there is little resistance and the nondominant hand moves in toward the chest, your energy is telling you to avoid that food.

This can also be done by holding a food or an object in your nondominant hand and following the steps of this testing method. An example I like to use is sugar. Hold a sugar cube in your nondominant hand and press firmly against it with your dominant hand. This is a processed, refined staple in most diets that rarely, if ever, is met with strong resistance.

Your body is capable of determining the nutritional energy you need to maintain a balance, if you allow it to communicate with you. It can also convey the areas of the internal body that might require the assistance of a physician.

To determine the efficiency or deficiency of your internal organs, you may use the same process. Call out your organs in sequence: liver, gallbladder, heart, small intestine, spleen, stomach, lung, large intestine, kidney, and bladder. This is also a pass/fail energy test. If any of the organs are deficient, your nondominant hand will have no resistance when you push firmly against it. A strong organ will produce a strong resistance, and the nondominant hand will remain tight and in position, three inches away from your chest in front of your heart.

The natural curative powers of body, mind, and spirit can be assisted by consciousness and superconscious nutritional diagnosis. However, there are times when we need the assistance of a physician who can guide us in the use of supplements, homeopathics, and other forms of natural healing that may include specific nutritional advice. When that is required, the EMT Surrogate Protocol can be of tremendous assistance to the diagnosing physician.

The EMT Surrogate Protocol

There are two significant factors regarding this protocol. First, it's an energy system. All living things, including humans and food, emit an electromagnetic energy. Not all energies are compatible. If you attend an evening party with fifty or so people, by the end of the night, you'll probably discover that you have made a series of great, good, not so good, and perhaps even bad connections. Such are the vicissitudes of life. The same is true with our relationship with various foods. Chances are pretty good that by the end of any given week, you will notice that some foods you ate during the week made a positive contribution to your overall health and well-being while others didn't. Everything is energy, and energy is infinitely diverse and exists in a constant state of flux. Not everything is compatible all of the time.

The second key factor regarding this diagnostic process is that, while we might not know it, we human beings are neurologically hardwired for a sixth sense. It's actually a part of our nervous system–generated bio-feedback loop, designed to provide us with a vigilant safety factor. Nature provides us with an added degree of heightened awareness whenever we're challenged as a part of our defense system. This vital process is engaged at a neuromuscular level.

Our nervous system is an extended network of transmission pathways, like a telecommunications grid that travels through the entire brain and body. Because this nerve network runs through the muscles, whenever we're confronted with any profound challenges or important questions, our brain initiates a cell-to-cell communication response between our brain and body via neuromuscular pathways. The most important brain centers that are engaged by this process are the stress centers, the hippocampus and the amygdala, as they determine and react to our perceived degree of safety. Thus, virtually any important questions we're confronted with trigger a response between our brain and body that is either a negative or a positive muscular reaction. Interestingly enough, the part of us that makes qualitative positive or negative judgment is our heart.

"The little brain within the heart" is where we're most capable of eliciting responses from within self. This is the place where our sixth-sensory awareness exercises its great intuitive power. Much more than just a mechanical region of deductive reasoning, this is a domain predominated by pure instinctive feeling. It's an area of hyper responsiveness that muscle testing can easily tap into.

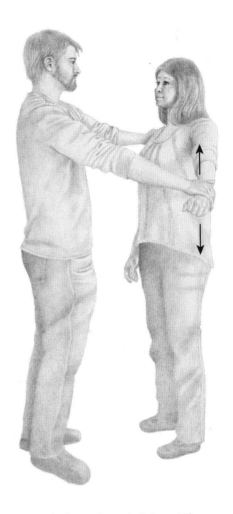

The process responds the same as PPF: a strong resistant muscle is reflective of a positive response, and a weak arm conveys a negative reaction.

The subject simply stands or sits in a comfortable position while the surrogate assistant and practitioner stand behind them. The surrogate assistant places one of their hands on the subject's shoulder. The surrogate's free arm (the test arm) should then rise to shoulder height.

First, the practitioner must conduct what's called an EMT (electomagnetic muscle testing) of the patient's organs and glands. This determines whether an organ or glandular system is imbalanced and specifically how. With energy, there are only three possible outcomes, excess, balanced, or deficient. There is also what we call a *causal root*, which should be determined by the practitioner. There may be several areas that are out of balance, but there is always one gland or one specific organ that is the root cause of the overall imbalance.

During EMT testing, the vital organs should be called out, one by one, as the practitioner simultaneously pushes down on the surrogate's arm. This happens while the surrogate's hand remains on the subject's shoulder.

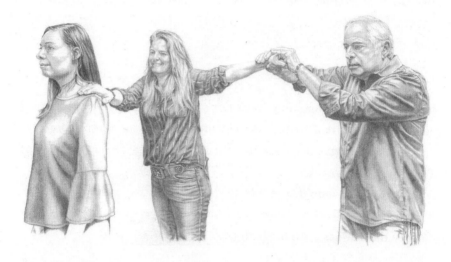

Thus, the surrogate is standing in as an energy proxy for the subject. If the surrogate's arm easily loses strength and goes down, it's a sign that the subject is channeling an energetic organ weakness through the surrogate's electromagnetic field. These weaknesses can be measured by degree through what I call pulse testing. By simply pulsing the surrogate's arm from one to ten, the practitioner can get a better idea as to just how overcharged or depleted the corresponding visceral imbalance is. The life force analysis (LFA) results are the primary determining factor for designing the subject's nutritional supplement plan.

Next, a list of foods should be verbally called out, one food at a time. As each food is being called out aloud, the practitioner should once again attempt to gently push down the surrogate's arm. Again, one of the surrogate's hands remains on the subject's shoulders. Thus, the intuition of the surrogate is determining the positive versus negative reactions to those foods that are being called out for the subject.

The subject has undergone an energetic LFA and food sensitivity test from which a detailed food list and nutritional supplement chart is compiled for them. Bio-energetic EMT nutrition testing is one of the most vital aspects of superconscious healing. It provides each patient with an energetically personalized map to direct them on their physical healing journey.

The Superconscious Healing Nutrition Plan

The superconscious healing nutrition plan begins with EMT food-sensitivity testing that enables us to identify those foods that our body has a difficult time digesting. Foods that are generally regarded as healthy and anti-inflammatory might not be when our body doesn't have the ability to recognize and assimilate them properly. Superconscious healing meal planning begins with engaging the EMT screening procedure in order to identify those foods most likely to trigger biochemical sensitivities.

Food Sensitivity Screening

The issue of food sensitivity is an emerging dilemma. As our food becomes ever more toxic, the result is an expanding list of food sensitivity related symptoms. Approximately 32 million Americans currently suffer from food allergies; that's nearly ten times the prevalence reported thirty-five years ago.[4]

I've seen a great number of patients diagnosed with virtually every disease and condition imaginable whose symptoms cleared up completely once they were able to diagnose and avoid food sensitivities. The proteins, carbohydrates, fats, and nutrients naturally occurring in foods can be unrecognizable inflammatory agents to the body. They can trigger reactions such as stomachaches, bloating, gas, bowel irregularities, headaches, hives, skin rashes, fatigue, shortness of breath, chest pain, swelling of bronchial passageway, anaphylaxis, insomnia, mood shifts, depression, and anxiety.

The most common allergenic sensitivity triggering foods are: dairy products, wheat, corn, shellfish, citrus, soy, peanuts, eggs, tomatoes, eggplant, peppers, and cabbage. Those are the common allergens, but anyone could be sensitive to virtually any food. The symptoms can be delayed for up to four days and can be as mild as a mood shift.

I've chosen to use the term *food sensitivity* to include both food allergies and food intolerances. There is, however, a big difference. Food intolerances present as generally non-life-threatening symptoms like rashes, stomachaches, and diarrhea and constipation, and they take place strictly within the digestive system.

Food allergies, on the other hand, represent potentially life-threatening symptoms such as anaphylaxis or dyspnea (the inability to breathe), and they occur within the immune system. Food allergies are very serious problems, and the problem is growing.

Food Sensitivity Avoidance

One of the most important aspects of food sensitivity testing is that it enables us to identify those foods that our body has a difficult time breaking down. Even those foods that are classified as anti-inflammatory become proinflammatory if our body doesn't have the ability to recognize and digest them. The reason the body may have a difficult time recognizing and breaking down certain foods is a lack of proper enzyme production.

Enzymes are catalysts that break down our foods into a more digestible state. According to *The Handy Biology Answer Book*, there are an estimated seventy-five thousand enzymes in the human body. The principal enzyme categories are: protease, which digests proteins; amylase, which digests carbohydrates (starches and sugars); and lipase, which digests fats.

The issue of food sensitivity is a growing problem in America. As we humans become increasingly stressed and impressionable and our food becomes ever more toxic, the result is an ever-growing correlative inflammatory symptomatology. Once a person has been EMT evaluated, a day-to-day meal plan can be constructed.

All foods belong to one of four major categories:

1. Proteins

2. Low-starch carbohydrates

3. High-starch carbohydrates

4. Low-glycemic fruits

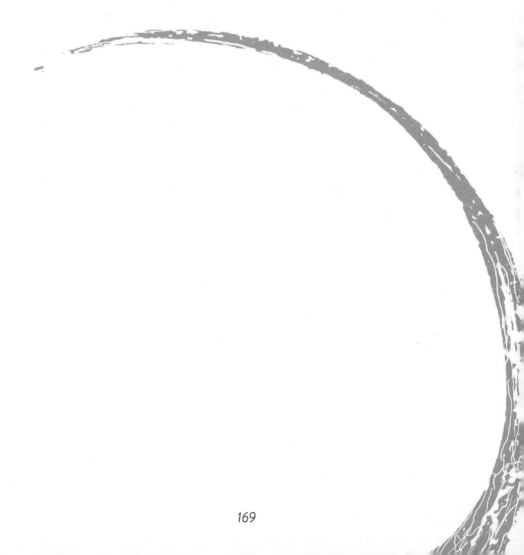

BAR CODED FOOD CHART

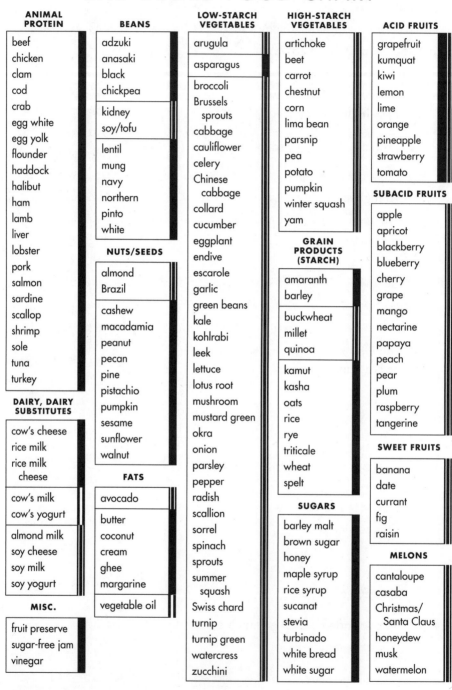

ANIMAL PROTEIN
- beef
- chicken
- clam
- cod
- crab
- egg white
- egg yolk
- flounder
- haddock
- halibut
- ham
- lamb
- liver
- lobster
- pork
- salmon
- sardine
- scallop
- shrimp
- sole
- tuna
- turkey

DAIRY, DAIRY SUBSTITUTES
- cow's cheese
- rice milk
- rice milk cheese
- cow's milk
- cow's yogurt
- almond milk
- soy cheese
- soy milk
- soy yogurt

MISC.
- fruit preserve
- sugar-free jam
- vinegar

BEANS
- adzuki
- anasaki
- black
- chickpea
- kidney
- soy/tofu
- lentil
- mung
- navy
- northern
- pinto
- white

NUTS/SEEDS
- almond
- Brazil
- cashew
- macadamia
- peanut
- pecan
- pine
- pistachio
- pumpkin
- sesame
- sunflower
- walnut

FATS
- avocado
- butter
- coconut
- cream
- ghee
- margarine
- vegetable oil

LOW-STARCH VEGETABLES
- arugula
- asparagus
- broccoli
- Brussels sprouts
- cabbage
- cauliflower
- celery
- Chinese cabbage
- collard
- cucumber
- eggplant
- endive
- escarole
- garlic
- green beans
- kale
- kohlrabi
- leek
- lettuce
- lotus root
- mushroom
- mustard green
- okra
- onion
- parsley
- pepper
- radish
- scallion
- sorrel
- spinach
- sprouts
- summer squash
- Swiss chard
- turnip
- turnip green
- watercress
- zucchini

HIGH-STARCH VEGETABLES
- artichoke
- beet
- carrot
- chestnut
- corn
- lima bean
- parsnip
- pea
- potato
- pumpkin
- winter squash
- yam

GRAIN PRODUCTS (STARCH)
- amaranth
- barley
- buckwheat
- millet
- quinoa
- kamut
- kasha
- oats
- rice
- rye
- triticale
- wheat
- spelt

SUGARS
- barley malt
- brown sugar
- honey
- maple syrup
- rice syrup
- sucanat
- stevia
- turbinado
- white bread
- white sugar

ACID FRUITS
- grapefruit
- kumquat
- kiwi
- lemon
- lime
- orange
- pineapple
- strawberry
- tomato

SUBACID FRUITS
- apple
- apricot
- blackberry
- blueberry
- cherry
- grape
- mango
- nectarine
- papaya
- peach
- pear
- plum
- raspberry
- tangerine

SWEET FRUITS
- banana
- date
- currant
- fig
- raisin

MELONS
- cantaloupe
- casaba
- Christmas/ Santa Claus
- honeydew
- musk
- watermelon

Alkaline Foods: Eat 4 for each 1 acid food.

Acid Foods: Eat 1 for every 4 alkaline foods.

Neutral Foods: These remain neutral only when your pH is stable.

Acid Foods: These convert to alkaline only when your pH is stable.

Superconscious Meal Planning

When setting up the superconscious meal plan, we want to lower our proinflammation levels, which means we must be very careful not to allow the ratio of high-starch carbohydrates to protein to exceed one to one (eating only one high-starch carb for every one protein). Most people who suffer from inflammation are considerably better off when the ratios of high-starch carbohydrates to protein are more like two to three (eating only two high-starch carbs for every three proteins). This is because starch and sugar require insulin for transport, and insulin is proinflammatory. When we consume a slightly higher ratio of protein to high starch carbohydrates, our body increases levels of the anti-inflammatory eicosanoid hormone glucagon. The superconscious meal plan is composed of three servings of protein; three servings of low-starch carbohydrates such as vegetables like zucchini, tomatoes, and broccoli; and only one to two servings per day of high-starch vegetables such as potatoes, corn, and beans.

Here is a sample meal plan:

BREAKFAST:
  Three or four organic egg whites with three-quarters cup of low-starch vegetables (see frittata recipe)

MIDMORNING SNACK:
  One serving of fruit

LUNCH:
  One cup of salad

  Three-quarters cup of protein (free-range poultry, wild fish, beans, legumes)

  Two tablespoons of monounsaturated oil (olive) with lemon juice

MIDAFTERNOON SNACK:

Two tablespoons of guacamole

Four tablespoons of sesame-free hummus (see hummus
bean dip recipe)

Three-quarters cup of celery or cucumber slices

DINNER:

Three-quarters cup of protein (free-range poultry, wild fish,
beans, legumes)

One cup of low-starch vegetables (asparagus, broccoli, green
beans, kale, spinach, zucchini)

One cup of high starch (brown rice, quinoa, potato, sweet
potato, winter squash)

Frittata Recipe

Breakfast is the most difficult meal for many of us because we have been
raised on excessively sweet, processed cereals. They are fast and easy
but not healthy. Instead, try egg white omelets or frittatas. They are
easier to make than most think, and the health and energy benefits
are tremendous.

Frittatas can be made on the stovetop or in the oven. Here is an easy
baked recipe for two people.

INGREDIENTS:

6 to 8 organic egg whites
1 ½ cup low-starch vegetables, finely chopped
1 teaspoon water
½ teaspoon olive oil or coconut oil (to grease the bottom
of the small baking dish)

INSTRUCTIONS:

Preheat the oven to 350 degrees. Sauté low-starch vegetables such as spinach, carrots, asparagus, mushrooms, or whatever else you want, and drain them of excess moisture. (You can use as many low-starch vegetables as you want, but I have found that limiting it to three distinct tastes is best.) Gently beat the egg whites together and slowly blend in the vegetables. Pour the mixture into an ovenproof baking dish. Bake for 20 to 25 minutes (keep an eye on it), until the eggs are puffed and appear cooked and the center of the frittata jiggles just a bit when you give it a gentle shimmy. Remove the frittata from the oven and place it on a cooling rack to cool. Garnish with herbs, slice with a sharp knife, and serve.

Easy Hummus without Tahini Recipe

This creamy hummus recipe requires just eight ingredients and five minutes to make. It's delicious, nutritious, and serves ten. Recipe courtesy of Hint of Joe's blog, October 27, 2014.

INGREDIENTS:

2 15-ounce cans of organic chickpeas (garbanzo beans), rinsed
2 cloves garlic
3 tablespoons olive oil
2 tablespoons fresh lemon juice
1 teaspoon cumin
¼ cup water
1 teaspoon salt
¼ teaspoon paprika

INSTRUCTIONS:

Add chickpeas, garlic, olive oil, lemon juice, cumin, water, and salt to a food processor. Blend until smooth and creamy (if needed, add more water one tablespoon at a time and continue blending until it

(Easy Hummus without Tahini Recipe, continued)

reaches your desired consistency). Transfer to a bowl. Sprinkle with paprika before serving.

Notes on hummus: For a smoother and creamier texture, remove the skins from the chickpeas by gently pinching them prior to step 1.

Any type of legume may be used in this recipe. Pinto beans or black beans make a wonderful bean dip.

Important Tips to Help Digestion

It is very important to avoid drinking while eating. The secretion of two enzymes, ptyalin and chyme, initiates digestion. They initiate the all-important five stages of digestion. If we drink during the meal, we run the risk of flushing, and thus diluting, the enzymes' vital digestive-triggering process. It's better to drink ninety minutes before or after eating.

I also recommend that virtually everybody take protease and amylase, which help break down carbohydrates and proteins, and lipase to help break down oils, fats, and triglycerides. These three enzymes should be taken immediately following each of the three major meals. Protease, amylase, and lipase Pure Formulas Enzyme Research brand is readily available via the internet.

Six Superconscious Healing Miracles

Six patients shared their stories of superconscious healing miracles to illustrate how important it is to determine the correct foods and nutritional supplements via energetic muscle testing. They all were in need of a practitioner to create a regimen for them because their disease was potentially life-threatening. Physicians and practitioners have an important role in the total health of their patients. When disease endangers a life, they are the knowledge source that can set up the framework of health for all aspects of body, mind, and spirit. However, it is up to the individuals to maintain the process to heal themselves.

These six individual experiences illustrate how important it is to determine the correct foods and nutritional supplements via energetic muscle testing. Recognizing the energetic conversation that goes on between our physical body and the foods and supplements we consume demonstrates the fullness of superconscious healing.

Laura's Miracle

Laura was a twenty-nine-year-old woman diagnosed with diminished ovarian reserves who worked with reproductive endocrinologists to correct her failed ovarian cycles. Her doctors found low thyroid, which is consistent with elevated antibodies. Her in vitro fertilization doctors considered Laura an anomaly, as medication didn't seem to help. At their peak, they were only able to produce seven eggs with two embryos.

After speaking to a friend, Laura decided to work with me through diet and supplements. After only three months on a gluten-free, dairy-free, anti-inflammatory diet bolstered by supplements, Laura's numbers were looking better, and she was feeling better as well. Following six months on the diet and the supplement program, Laura was producing seventeen eggs with ten embryos. Shortly thereafter, Laura was thrilled to find out that she was pregnant. Her endocrinologists were absolutely stunned, and I'm happy to report that Laura now has two beautiful children.

Patrick's Miracle

Patrick was diagnosed with sudden hearing loss as part of an autoimmune sensory condition. Doctors initially put him on steroids for four years. At first the medication worked. But, as time went by, it was less effective and eventually stopped working all together. When Patrick asked, "Where do we go from here?" he was told he had to live with it. He was told to get hearing aids and that there was nothing that could be done.

A friend referred him to me, and I performed an extensive question-and-answer session and a series of muscle tests where I discovered he had a lymphatic deficiency, spleen inflammation, adrenal exhaustion, and environmental allergies to mold. Following a three-month anti-inflammatory diet that was yeast free, combined with supplements supporting his deficient organ systems, Patrick had 90 to 100 percent hearing restored with no need for hearing aids.

Corina's Miracle

In 2009, Corina began having vision problems to the extent that she lost her vision completely. She also suffered from severe headaches. Her doctor performed an MRI and discovered that she had meningioma tumor the size of a walnut in her brain. The doctor told her that she would require surgery to remove the tumor and that there were two different ways in which this might be accomplished. One way was through the nose, and the other was to open her skull. Due to the size of her tumor, the doctors were forced to go through her skull. She experienced a successful surgery; her headaches were gone, and her vision once again returned. She was healthy for one year; then once again her symptoms returned, and an MRI revealed that the tumor had grown back.

She was determined not to have a second surgery; that was when she came to see me. I muscle tested her extensively, tested her organs and glands, and checked for food allergies. I adjusted her diet on a monthly basis, and eventually her headaches disappeared and her vision drastically improved. She remained on the diet and two years later was 100 percent tumor free. Corina has remained tumor free for nine years.

Erin's Miracle

In 1996, while Erin and her family were on a ski vacation, she felt a hard lump in her breast. She went to see her doctor, who diagnosed her with breast cancer. He recommended a lumpectomy followed by chemotherapy for six months and radiation for three months. After six months of chemotherapy, Erin was weak, nauseous, and suffering extreme hair loss; her spirit was depleted. In her words, she was "a walking dead person." She simply couldn't go through chemo or radiation anymore.

A neighbor referred her to me. She was amazed to discover that we were not only working toward a stronger body—we were also working with her energy and spirit. Erin described herself as a sugar-holic, so I immediately began implementing a program to support her pH and to change her diet. We also did a hair analysis to check mineral patterns. At that point, Erin felt she was improving and went on another family ski trip, only this time she felt strong enough to go skiing. She realized she was recovering from her cancer. After only two short weeks on her diet and supplement plan, she began feeling healed and self-empowered. In her words, she was "finally awakened to life." Her doctors confirmed that her cancer was no more.

In 2015, Erin was diagnosed with osteoporosis from the previous chemo. She returned to my office and brought her bone density tests. Her physicians told her that she needed medication to stop the bone loss, and she was told explicitly that it was not possible to grow new bone. After a year on the diet and supplement plan, she improved her osteoporosis to osteopenia. She continued taking her supplements and staying on her diet for two years; she had another bone density test that confirmed she had grown all of her bone back. She no longer has osteoporosis, and she has been cancer free for twenty-two years.

Adriano's Miracle

Eight years ago, Adriano began stumbling, tripping over his own feet and falling down. He was diagnosed with Parkinson's disease. In addition, he was thirty pounds overweight. His doctors put him on medication, which helped only a little bit. His condition continued to swiftly progress, and his worst symptom was that he couldn't swallow. Due to the fact that his brother was diagnosed with Parkinson's and his disease had advanced even with pharmaceutical drugs, Adriano was anxious and felt he had to take some other form of action. A friend referred him to me; I immediately performed muscle tests and discovered he had inflammation and most of his symptoms were triggered by a retrovirus. I put him on antiviral supplements and an anti-inflammatory diet. In only twenty-one days, his movement became fluid and strong. In addition, he lost thirty pounds and improved his fitness by walking three miles three times a week. His neurologists were in total disbelief, and Adriano is now relatively symptom free.

Lisa's Miracle

Lisa was a very sick child who spent a lot of time in a children's hospital. She was diagnosed as a pre-diabetic with pancreatitis and atypical cystic fibrosis.

Her mother had heard about me from a friend, and when she first came to see me, I performed muscle testing. I put her on a strict diet and supplemental regime. At first, she was a bit reluctant to follow my program, but as fate would have it, she had a pancreatic attack that was serious enough to require hospitalization. This experience made her decide to follow the program more strictly. After two years, her blood sugars are normal, her pancreatitis no longer exists, and concerning her atypical cystic fibrosis, she is asymptomatic. In addition, Lisa has grown spiritually out of this experience and learned to become more dedicated to her wholeness.

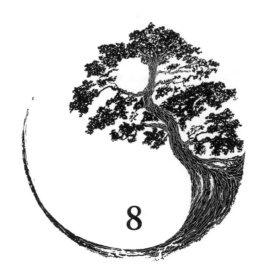

8

Superconsciousness

What happens when you make the dynamic shift from material limitation to miracle-making enlightenment? From personal experience and
hundreds of client cases I know that what happens is superconscious
healing!

We've explored the various aspects of consciousness and superconsciousness, but there are Three Integral Objectives and Five Cardinal
Tenets that can help you achieve the ultimate goal of superconscious healing. I'm not suggesting that these principles need to be followed with rigid,
devotional exactitude; rather, I feel that the general spirit of their message
needs be embraced by our deepest intent. That alone should be more than
enough to inspire the natural elevation to superconsciousness, especially
when combined with the consistent practice of prayer, meditation, and
trance manifest.

It's likely that each of the following axioms will translate as something uniquely different to every person who reads them. That's fine, because superconscious healing is about dedicating ourselves to the progressive uplifting of our mindful awareness. These axioms are designed to inspire and provide a path for those seekers who wish to find direction from within the deepest depths of your own sacred source.

The Three Integral Objectives

The Three Integral Objectives help us to be more mindful and aware of our wholeness. They are:

1. To Realize Our Immortality

2. To Illuminate Our Divine Wisdom

3. To Access Our Unlimited Power

To Realize Our Immortality, the first integral objective, may be taken either figuratively or literally.

If you are an agnostic, you might prefer to think of it as an allegory. Instead of being asked to awkwardly ponder the question of your immortality from a spiritual perspective, you might find it more comfortable to look at it from the standpoint of energy. Everything visible, as well as that which is not seen by the physical eye, is composed of energy. Each of us is energy, and as Einstein stated, energy can neither be created nor destroyed. Energy expands, and it contracts, but it never dissipates. Beyond the material manifestation of energy we perceive as reality, we are composed of energetic properties that are indestructible, and since we are manifestations of energy, we live on and on, transmuting from one manifestation to another. That energy is the immortality that needs to be recognized.

From a metaphysical perspective, we eternally evolve in spirit to travel the progressive path of karmic lessons to the goal of dharmic enlightenment. In this case, spirit is the energy that continues throughout perpetuity. From this point of view, the spirit is the energy of immortality.

Regardless of the method used to define it, both perspectives reach the realization of immortality. No matter which view is most comfortable for you, it's time to pursue the more personal questions, like:

"Who exactly am I?"

"Who and what do I see when I gaze into my own eyes while looking into the mirror?"

From a material standpoint, the answer to both is simple: you are what you see in physical form. Expand the depth of your search and ask yourself these questions:

"What is the unseen life force that flows within my cells, tissues, and organs?"

"What animates my being?"

"What makes the difference within me between life and death?"

Even though many hold a belief in the eternal soul, much of the Western world still struggles to grasp an understanding of their own immortality. For the most part, there is no cultural knowledge base that teaches us how to identify with such an esoteric concept. That's partially because Western culture is profoundly adept at surviving in the physical realm. Material living represents the baseline of our existence. This is who we think we are. We worship the human physical form and relate to success based on the material trappings that surround the physical form. Spiritual references of immortality are becoming more common but, in many arenas, conversations on the topic are still awkward. We haven't been educated in understanding that we are more than we perceive in the third dimension. It can be difficult to expose ourselves to the unseen realities of the multiverse because realizing one's immortality requires a thorough and honest examination of self. Understanding the validity of the perpetual continuation of the soul might seem like a massive breakthrough in consciousness to some of us. In fact, it is. But the acceptance of immortality is integral to superconsciousness.

Miracles demand a higher state of awareness that emanates from the immortal self, and they can't be expected to appear when restriction is imposed by mortal limitations. If we release that constraint and view the soul without imposing any boundaries, we can reveal the power that exists within us. When we consciously connect with the eternal soul that peers back at us when we gaze into a mirror, we accept the awareness that we are the reflection of our limitless source.

The cultivation of the process, unlike what we're accustomed to in the physical realm, does not entail doing more to achieve the goal. It's actually about doing less to arrive at a state of pure being-ness. It's about letting go of the monkey mind, a Buddhist term that means "restless and confused." We need to abandon and release these so that we may allow ourselves to tap into our true immortal being-ness.

The second integral objective, To Illuminate Our Divine Wisdom, can help filter the quantity and quality of useless information we are bombarded with daily so that we may access our immortal self and adopt a permanent meditative presence.

The sheer volume of information we process during an average day is truly astronomical. Considering this deluge of data, one must ask: "What am I actually hearing? And how does it influence or shape my life?"

Some of what we hear is positive, some is negative, some comes from thought centers deep within us, some is rife with confusion and uncertainty, and some is determined and uplifting. Some of what is heard is the echoes of voices other than our own. These may be voices from our present or from our past, voices of friends or voices of enemies, loving voices, and even voices of abuse.

Unfortunately, the ever-expanding bombardment of dark information from every imaginable source has disrupted our vibrational stability to such an extent that a twenty-minute meditation is not adequate to counterbalance the negative unconscious mind. The totality of this results in shifting and unstable moods and a complete disconnect from the universal mind.

Ask yourself, How much of what I hear can be classified as elevating and healing? How much is reflective of true wisdom? The value of what we hear comes through filtering and consciously screening all the subconscious or unconscious noise because what we absorb ranges from divine to dangerous.

This screening process demands conscious proactive thought instead of subconscious or unconscious reactive thought. The application of conscious proactive thought initiates the practice of tapping into and regulating the stream of information that becomes our reality. Once again, we need to be the observer. This time we need to monitor and inspect information we receive and the manner in which we process it. Just as with meditation and trance, this is part of the development needed to connect with divine universal wisdom.

By exercising the active states of choice and discernment, we intentionally select what information we receive and value with every thought. It requires consciously moving beyond the typical busy-mindedness of day-to-day life. Mindful awareness of the thoughts that enter your brain and heart help you enter a state of waking meditation.

This awareness affects much more than the personal mind; it's much more vast. It's the Universal mind of which we are a part. As we achieve a greater competence in waking meditation, we naturally become more unified with the Universal mind. That connection permits a clear path to divine wisdom, for the Universal mind is the source of all divine wisdom.

The third integral objective, To Access Our Unlimited Power, is the culmination of bringing the first two objectives together. Miracles demand power and not just any power. Miracles demand power that knows no limits.

In many ways, the three integral objectives are sequentially interdependent. Only by realizing our immortality and illuminating our Divine wisdom can we generate and gain access to unlimited power. Any discussion about our immortality and our Divine wisdom implies the kind of preeminence that can only be invoked by the soul, the spirit, and the Universal mind. These transcendent domains of our self represent our natural places of higher power.

Energy innately flows from these dynamic centers, and it knows no limit. The formula is accumulation of energy equals power. The more intensified the energy, the greater its power. In most cases, it's about allowing energy to flow and assemble into power without interruption or obstruction.

Many of us want to increase power in various aspects of our lives, but we often end up getting in the way of our own flow. We impede our progress by building dams of confusion and uncertainty. In essence, it's just as crucial to stay out of power's way as it is to generate power.

Humans tend to sabotage personal power by doubting their ability. Instead, we should reinforce it with expectancy because expectancy of our unlimited power helps to make it a reality. The energy we infuse into confidence kindles the flame of manifest action. It's less a matter of tapping into unlimited power and more about generating it through positive thinking. The only thing that can truly weaken our ability to generate personal power is the lack of belief in it and in ourselves.

If you subscribe to the old axiom "seeing is believing," you might want to take a closer look at your relationship with self-doubt. However, if you support the principle that "believing is seeing," you have probably already accessed your unlimited power.

The Five Cardinal Tenets

A tenet is a guiding philosophy. It's little life lesson that might seem a bit pretentious, but the knowledge gained from it forms the foundation of a greater understanding of self and all of the dimensional realities we inhabit. Tenets inherently inspire and guide us in a more enlightened direction. The Five Cardinal Tenets are:

1. To Know "The Way": To understand the knowledge of natural law and to harmoniously participate in the flow of life from birth through growth, to death and rebirth

2. To Embrace the Whole: To live in accord with "the whole" and to know that the darkness exists in perfect, mutual compatibility with the light

3. To Balance Energy: To become a master of energy and to live in rapport with the fluid interchange between energy and matter

4. To Flow from Source: To emanate from the core of our immortal soul

5. To Expand the Mind: To cultivate higher consciousness and to ultimately merge with Universal mind

To Know "The Way"

Aligning with the natural order and maintaining mindfulness governs and enlivens the substance and activity of all things. Accessing super-consciousness via waking mediation is the beginning of a lifestyle change—a lifestyle of higher consciousness by learning to harmonize with The Way.

The Way is what ancient Taoist sages called, the *Hsien t'ien chih-ch'i*; it roughly translates to "primordial energy that existed even before creation." It is the beginning, the middle, and the end. It is the most fundamental path—a path of zero resistance where only the empty hand can be filled full and only the empty handed can be fulfilled.

The tenet of The Way isn't just any old way. It is *THE* Way. It animates and governs the movement of all and everything and is deeply rooted in the very core of superconscious healing. The Way is about blending with the unseen force that conducts the living symphony of life. It's a symphony that crescendos and de-crescendos in endless swells of creation and destruction. Even the disorder of its decay is reflective of its greater harmony as it endlessly gives birth to a continuum of reorganization. The Way is as elusive as it is compelling. It cannot be envisaged by a callous heart nor seen through the jaded eye.

It's an elusive life-governing source that gives direction to all and everything in the infinite universe. It's elusive because The Way cannot be grasped by the mortal senses. The Way can't be deciphered by the ordinary mind; it can only be clarified by the Universal mind. By observing, decoding, and adhering to the natural physics of The Way, we align ourselves with Universal consciousness and, in so doing, harness ourselves to our own limitless source.

The Way is the gossamer cord that threads together infinite being-ness. It divulges the imponderable *how* of all things, both seen and unseen. It's the innate intelligence that awakens all to the harmonic rhythms of life. It's the choreography of the Universe in its infinite cosmic dance of life.

The Way enlivens and directs all energy, subtle and great, and reflects the everlasting whole-ism of which everything is bound together. It is a mirror of the integral Universe that surrounds us and the internal Universe that courses deep within our being.

Due to the cause and effect of The Way, every thought and willful act aligns with either flow or resistance. When we are living in balance, we flow. When we are living out of balance, we meet with resistance. This represents the continuity of whole-ism. Whether we fall or we rise is up to us. I like to think that the Universe gives us two options, lessons or blessings. Flow represents blessing, and resistance is all about lessons. Ultimately, the blessings of flow and the lessons of resistance end up in the same positive place of enlightenment.

To Embrace the Whole

Wholeness is reflective of The Way of things. Thus, The Way is all-inclusive. We are all part of a unified whole. Separation is not part of The Way of things. Rather, it is an illusion.

Thousands of years ago, ancient Taoist sages deciphered natural laws that were believed to hold the secret to living a life of integral balance. One of these canons states that all antagonisms are complementary and goes so far as to posit that opposites represent two components of the same source. Those Taoists clearly understood and appreciated that the natural opposition of duality represented a paradox whereby all opposites balanced each other out.

The entire symphony of life is a harmonious blending of opposing energies. If we examine the opposing powers of nature, we see that they blend and harmonize in accordance with a higher purpose. Mighty hurricanes naturally defoliate the earth, clearing the way for the birthing of a new generation of vegetation. Exposing the human body to a safe, allowable presence of germs ultimately strengthens the immune system. It's not possible to pry apart the opposition from the harmony, as they are both vital aspects of one whole synergy.

The harmony of opposition presents us with a considerable challenge, for we've been raised on a steady diet of black and white, and the shades of gray are overlooked. There's much more to life than winning or losing, and losing alone could never be as damaging as living in a state of mind where the two are believed to be separate from each other. We've been told to believe we exist in a polarized environment of one good side and one bad side. It's our affliction that carries us from light to dark and back again, leaving us the victims of ever-changing conditions from one moment to the next. I call this half-ness. Half-ness separates the good from the bad and rejects the bad completely. In so doing, it disempowers. In contrast, wholeness is an empowering concept that generates its strength from inclusiveness.

The primordial Tai Chi circle, or yin-yang symbol, represents a synergistic image of balance and wholeness. It personifies the duality in the multiverse, good and bad, light and dark, happy and sad, etc. It speaks to an unbroken mutual compatibility of opposition. You can't separate the good from the bad, the darkness from the light, the happiness from the sadness, etc. Both extremes are equally necessary components of one perfect whole. In no way is their opposing presence purely inflexible, because they signify so much more than just a static yin-yang symbol. They actually represent the most stimulated dynamic energy of the multiverse. The sacred tension imparted between the two extremes gives birth to an eternal dance where each opposite power is forever simultaneously pouring itself into and becoming the other.

Most of us are inclined to embrace the good, the light, and the happiness side of the dualistic equation. We turn away from the bad, the dark, and the sadness. By favoring the positive over the negative, we not only separate ourselves from the unpleasant, we separate ourselves from a wholeness that includes our very selves. There's a dynamic tension between all dualistic extremes that generates a unifying natural power. The whole is always greater than the sum of its parts. There is no power in half-ness.

We have been conditionally trained to believe that life is good only when all material conditions have been favorably met. As long as money and love are in abundance in our lives, everything appears to be fine. We are inclined to think difficulties and problems represent bad days. Wholeness consciousness understands the delicate, yet vital, interconnection between the obvious benefit of a good day and the potential benefit of a bad day. This kind of synergistic appreciation prevents one from giving a day a negative rating for whatever reason.

Maybe it's raining. To embrace the wholeness of that rainy day, we might consider the fact that the rain is nourishing our vegetable garden and cleaning the air. Wholeness provides a knowledge and understanding that every negative experience is always, in some way, producing a positive experience. At the time, we may not recognize that the end result is favorable, but when one exists in superconscious wholeness, we know the final outcome will be constructive because opposing cycles create each other and ultimately manifest in wholeness.

Think about it this way: every victory you've ever celebrated in your life is directly tied to and the result of every previous loss. By understanding and embracing wholeness, we gain access to its infinite power—power that can only result when we free ourselves from the torment of the endless ups and downs.

How do we perceive ourselves? Are we whole or un-whole? Is the lens of self that we project our life through perceived by us as integrated or dis-integrated? Are the two coherent or chaotic? Do we feel as though we part of a bigger picture, such as family, neighborhood, community, nation, world, and universe? Do we even fit into our own picture? Can we unconditionally accept and love the partially flawed duality that makes up our "whole" self?

There is no question that we're all inextricably bound to a greater whole-ism. The larger question is about our personal wholeness. Do you feel a sense of connectedness, power, and purpose in your life? Do you feel a balance and alignment between the outer world and your inner world? When we're separated from the whole, we are powerless. Superconscious living and healing depend on our ability to link to the unlimited power of wholeness. To more fully align our superconscious frame of mind, we must learn to cultivate a mentality that transcends all distorted thinking about the adversarial illusion of separation.

The most powerful natural law that embodies superconscious healing is called the mutual compatibility of opposition. This law begins with the understanding that the outcome of every action results in a dualistic possibility. Here in the West, we tend to think of opposites as qualitatively antagonistic. For most of us, the result is either good or bad. We see it as two forces engaged in a tug of war against one another, resulting in an outcome where one dominates the other. Most of us fail to grasp the elusive lesson in all this. But what seems to be a puzzling paradox is really just opposites that are dynamically interdependent. Each of the two extremes make up one half of a complete whole. The duality as seen by The Way of things isn't good or bad; instead it is either wholeness or half-ness.

The more one contemplates this enlightened perspective, the greater is its empowering wisdom. Think of a difficult situation currently in your life. Chances are you're focused on the final result as either good or bad. Don't get too distracted by the words *good* and *bad*. The key word here is the word *or*. You see, there is no *or* because the word *or* connotes half of the whole. *Or* is merely an illusion, for the Universe is unquestionably whole.

A deeper look into The Way of things reveals a creational relationship between opposites. If you continue to pour water into a pitcher, the same action that filled the pitcher up will eventually force it to spill out over the brim. Filling up eventually results in emptying out. This creational relationship between opposites is in evidence in all aspects of life. Everything is created by the interwoven elements of opposition. The same holds true for the sacred tension between the good and the bad in day-to-day life. All the variables that make up the difficult processes that challenge us are part of one experience. It's impossible to separate the darkness of our problems from the light of their solutions. Separateness is a powerful illusion that, ironically, can only serve to separate us from The Way, for the Universe is about order rather than randomness. Creational duality is a very important part of the Universal order. It's not about one thing or the other. It's about one thing and the other. Most importantly, it's about two opposite motions working together in syncopated piston-like fashion to create flow.

While I was writing my second book, *The Tao of Ch'i*, in 1992, I suffered with the greatest writer's block I've ever experienced. I was a third of the way into the book when my brother died. The tragedy of his passing cast a pall over my life, but it also opened my heart in a way that influenced some of the most inspired writing I've ever done. Because of that experience, I find it unnatural, if not impossible, to separate pain from inspiration. There have been many other dark periods in my life that, not so surprisingly, reinforced the very same lesson.

As is always the case, the Universe knew exactly what it was doing every step of the way. I've come to believe that each and every one of us is confronted with precisely what we need, and it's probably precisely what we asked for in the spirit realm before we were conceived. The underlying value is that with the pain and suffering there comes a transcendent liberation. Opposites are forever creating each other and ultimately reveal the perfectly imperfect wholeness.

Difficult situations tear us down in some ways, even as they simultaneously build us up in other ways. It's a question of having faith in the wholeness, an understanding and trust in a natural process that knows exactly when and how we need to have an old domain leveled to the foundation and a new structure erected. It's a type of surrender of personal will to the way of universal wisdom.

The act of surrender brings up many questions. Do we feel safe surrendering our fate to the mutual compatibility of opposition? If the Universe has everything under control, should we even bother trying to engage our will, and if so, when? Is it possible for us to positively affect our life journey during a difficult period? Do we have the ability to manifest change and affect the dual possibility of outcomes?

We do have a choice in the matter. The mutual compatibility of opposition is a law as fixed as fate meaning the universe always has the last word in all outcomes. But don't forget that as long as you cultivate superconsciousness, you are the Universe! By both surrendering to the predestined will of the Universe and knowing your path is in alignment with The Way of things, you are the Universe. Harmonize superconsciousness with the unblemished wisdom of the Universe and know that you are part of that wholeness!

Think back in your life and retrieve a memory of an event that you perceived as negative. Perhaps your focus settles on a time when you were released from a job or demoted or experienced a failed relationship. As time and the pain of the event passed, did you find a better position, expand your horizons, or find new relationships? There is always a new opportunity that surfaces from what might be viewed as negative, but it is important how you adapt to the concept that good and bad are two parts of the same energy that bring value to the whole.

Next, think about how you would react to something that was not constructive to your present-day life. Can you step back from it with the knowledge that the emptiness or void is about to be filled with something productive or beneficial? That understanding is part of the expectancy of wholeness that threads through our lives. The adage "When one door closes, another opens" is also the way the Universe flows.

It's easy to understand why any assertions of Universal wholeness are countered with cynicism and doubt. Looking at the troubled world we exist in, it's hard not to feel enveloped in chaos and confusion. What we may consider bad or negative seems to always be the focus of life. The feeling of oppression disassociates us from others and from ourselves. Life in our world is anything but whole; at least that's how it appears on the surface.

Patient stories reflect similar disturbing pictures of dis-unity and fragmentation. When we look around us, there's a tendency to feel as though we're living in a universe overcome with darkness. The human mind is prone to be trapped in an illusionary vacuum of separation. We've not been taught, nor are humans inclined, to see good and bad as an integrated whole. But there does exist an extrinsic and an intrinsic duality that is always at work in the Universe. Recognize and know that discord is aligned with order. That which may appear shattered on the surface remains ever connected to a deeper unbroken whole at its core. Opposites are not inseparable. They are interdependent. Together they represent wholeness because only the maximum darkness can provide the sharpest contrast for the brightest of light.

Entanglement perfectly describes a Universe where everything is unified and engaged in the unceasing action of creation. It's a cosmic dance that began with a big bang 13.8 billion years ago when all manifestations of energy were set into a perpetual motion of endless change and evolution. The Universe is alive and unified by much more than subatomic particles and smaller elementary particles. It is a living Universe that is undivided and animated by consciousness. Consciousness gives rise to matter. It's pervasive. It is the binding life force, the foundation of the Universe, that is present in every particle. It is the reason why something that appears to be shattered on the surface remains forever connected to a deeper unbroken whole at its core. It's called self-transcendence.

Self-transcendence is a state where the ego perspective of self vanishes, and in its place, a far greater Universal concept of self emerges. It's also the simultaneous transcendence of our un-whole self and the occupation of the highest level of our undivided self.

Researching self-transcendence is a growing trend. A fascinating Johns Hopkins study once looked at how a group of terminally ill subjects responded to the prospect of facing imminent death. The research team, headed by psychiatrist Roland Griffiths, wanted to see whether or not the psychedelic properties of psilocybin, a drug often used in brain research, might help end-stage cancer patients confront death with a greater sense of wholeness. After the trial, many of the subjects of this study reported that they had been deeply moved by the experience. Some described the feeling as a powerful merger with the Divine. They went on to describe it as unification with the greater whole that gave them a transformative sense of belonging that they had never before experienced.[1]

Contemporary psychiatric science defines these self-transcendant states as peak moments when people feel uplifted beyond the humdrum of everyday life and they feel profoundly connected to the greater whole. In such states, many people often report feeling an empowering sense that arises from the communion.

This state does not have to be achieved via a drug. There are a number of studies that show our natural ability to activate similar areas of the brain through meditation, trance, and mindfulness. However it is achieved, self-transcendence represents an otherworldly aspect of the human experience capable of radically altering the reality base line.

Throughout history, humans have lifted themselves up and into modes of self-transcendence through various rituals. The common denominator is an altered consciousness that elevates us above our ordinary mind and transports us beyond the everyday mental processes to a more magical, mystical mentality.

What is going on when we're in the state of self-transcendence, and what is the significance of it?

Technically, neural plasticity research indicates that self-transcendence tends to decrease activity in the brain's posterior superior parietal lobe. That acts as the GPS system in the brain and helps distinguish the boundaries of self in space, identifying it as separate from everything else. By reducing activity in this area, the brain can no longer separate itself from the surrounding environment, which results in a greater sense of immersive unification. Research has also discovered that modes of self-transcendence markedly increase the brain's production of the peptide hormone oxytocin, which is often referred to as "the love drug." It increases our natural drive to bond. Typically secreted during stress free periods, it promotes powerful feelings of togetherness and tranquility.

We can create this same total access via thought alone. Energizing the manner in which we think can propagate brain changes capable of radically altering the relativity of our reality. Mind changes brain. Brain changes body. Together they alter actuality.

The mental catalysts of meditation, trance, and mindfulness precipitate change and represent the most powerful manifestations of conscious proactive thought. Engaging the power of our mind, we can transcend the illusion of un-whole self because superconscious healing embraces whole-ism unconditionally.

Most of us are unaware of it, but we're all born with a natural attraction to suffering. Darkness that surfaces in the form of pain and suffering is part of a whole that includes light. In the final analysis we must remember: the destination of all pain and suffering is peace.

Superconscious growth and evolution are energized by a unease that arises between our darkness and light. In our darkness, there is pain and suffering that results from willful resistance. Our light, however, represents living in flow and culminates with liberation.

If our wrong choices hurt badly enough and last long enough, they'll likely generate a greater desire for peace. That's powerful enough to inspire what the Buddha called "right living." This is the Universe's way of softening our willful egos. This is the value of transitioning from the will of our ego to will of the Universe.

The beauty of superconscious wholeness is that in order to be truly whole, it must include suffering and peace, as well as karma and dharma. Ironically, it's our attraction to suffering that masses spiritual pain that ultimately ushers the path of our liberation. The great paradox of wholeness is unmistakable; separation is an illusion, even the separation between our suffering and our peace. You simply cannot have one without the other. To have the peace without the pain is un-whole. As with all other paradoxical dualities, there exists an indelible mutual compatibility of opposition.

Whenever we look hopelessly at the circumstances surrounding our pain, our tendency is to narrow our vision to a microcosmic perspective and view the hurt and suffering in our lives as a misfortune. If we fail to take a step back and view our pain and suffering from a macrocosmic perspective, we violate our own sense of completeness, which only serves to perpetuate our suffering.

In order for us to spiritually evolve beyond the continuation of our own mortal limitations, we must come to accept the fact that the universe is orderly, especially in the midst of chaos. Many of us view ourselves as the arbiters of universal order and justice. If it doesn't go the way we want, we chalk it up as chaos. But every lesser disorder is a necessary and a vital part of the greater order. Without disorder, there could be no order. Every polarity is forever blending into its opposite, and every opposite is merging back into its opposition in a never-ending cosmic dance.

When we observe our karmic pain, we believe we are looking into darkness, but the darkness we think we see is nothing more than an illusion. What we are truly looking at is an inseparable whole that includes the true nature of our precious self. The superconscious mind knows well that in order to become the miracle that creates miracles, we must first unconditionally embrace the dark illusion of wholeness.

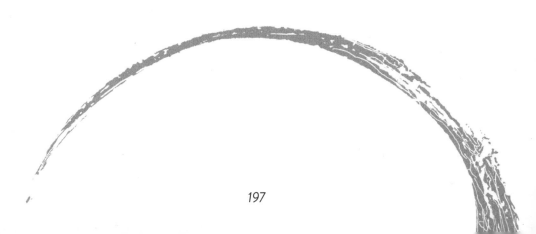

To Balance Energy

The Superconscious Eight Laws of Energy establish the foundation of the superconscious evolution from matter-centric consciousness to energy-centric consciousness.

1. Reality Begins at the Energy Level: Quantum mechanics tells us that everything is composed of 99.999 percent energy. Einstein said that energy and matter are interconvertible and transferrable. We are energy. Our thoughts are energy. Our intentions are energy. Our emotions are energy. Our words are energy. Our food is energy. Our places of habitation are energy. Everything is energy!

2. Energy Is Unified: Separation is an illusion. The ancient Taoists taught that the Universe is enlivened and unified by energy. They subscribed to a unified theory that links all energies cosmologically. Matter depicts an illusion of divided detachment. Energy is the unifying power.

3. Energy Can Neither Be Created nor Destroyed: Being-ness is infinite and ever changing. Death pertains only to the material realm. Energy is everlasting through its many changing manifestations. It is infinitely interchangeable. Cells are destructible. Fields, particles, and atoms are indivisible and indestructible. They can only be rearranged, and repositioned.

4. The Snowflake Law (energy is unique, or sui generis): Even though all manifestations of energy are unified by the same source, like snowflakes, each is unique. At the energetic level, all living things have a unique DNA-like constitution. This is an especially important point when it comes to healing. No two forms of any given disease, health condition, or prescriptions are exactly the same from one patient to the next. Every form of diabetes, heart disease, and lung cancer may carry the same material label, but each is energetically unique. Also, every person is unique, and each patient is going to respond to his or her condition and treatment in their own way. I have had patients who could only effectively kill antibiotic resistant strep bacteria with twenty grams of vitamin C per day, while other patients experienced acute attacks of diarrhea with as little as one five hundred milligram dose of vitamin C.

5. Energy Is in a Constant State of Flux: The Way reminds us that adaptation precedes transformation; this is key to healing and personal growth. Everything is constantly changing. Nothing stays the same. Static systems of medicine and healing fail to anticipate change and are therefore ineffective. In order for healthcare systems to be truly effective, they must be able to anticipate patterns of change in order to effectively execute disease prevention. Energy results as an excess (overflow), balance (flow), or deficiency (lack). I often test a patient for a food like blueberries, and they pass the test. They then proceed to eat blueberries nearly every day for several months. When they return for follow up testing, they fail the energy muscle test for blueberries. Failure to rotate one's diet causes an energy imbalance of excess.

6. All Manifestations of Energy Share One Source: All energy is unified at the source level. All things spring forth from and are animated by one source. Separation is an illusion. Energy flows when it emanates from source. Energy is resistant when it fails to remain aligned with source. Flow results as balance. Resistance results as an imbalance (excess or deficiency) of energy. Maintaining connectivity with source is essential for sustained balance, ease and wholeness.

7. Every Energetic Imbalance Has a Causal Root: This is an extremely important matter when it comes to medicine and healing. For example, a patient diagnosed with kidney disease may be causally rooted in a faulty digestive system that fails to produce the proteolytic enzymes necessary to digest protein. Undigested food proteins might then deposit in the kidneys, causing inflammation. Thus, the kidneys are not the direct cause of this inflammatory problem, poor protein digestion is. This demonstrates how energy sequences through cause and effect; there is a causal root to trigger systemic health problems. Mainstream allopathic medicine and pharmaceutical medicine clearly have their place. But there can be no doubt that the world is in dire need of effective energy-based medicines and protocols that go beyond the application of side-effect-causing medicinal bandages. It is far better that we get to the systemic root of our health problems, especially for purposes of disease prevention.

The main point of medicine is to heal and, at the very least, to do no harm. Currently, one hundred thousand Americans die from prescription drugs each year; that's 270 per day—more than twice as many as are killed in automobile accidents.[2]

8. Matter Is Altered at the Energetic Level: Energy generates vibration that represents a myriad of frequencies. Some frequencies produce balance; some produce imbalance. A simple loving touch can produce a balancing frequency. Every food, every vitamin, every sip of water, and every thought (stressful and/or peaceful) produces varying vibrational frequencies that alter matter.

Energy and matter represent relativity that is made up of two parts as one whole. From ancient times to the present, every world culture has established a reality baseline that was predominantly energy based or matter based. Societies program their masses to understand life from the bias of their mainstream cultural perspective. The ancient Eastern cultural experience based its reality on energy. Our modern Western cultural experience is reality based on matter. In terms of reality, our five senses betray us, as the science of physics has established that everything is energy. This fact is extremely significant for superconscious evolution. Virtually everything superconscious healing espouses to, from its manifest exercises to its diagnostics and nutritional therapies, is energy based. The very foundation of is reality is rooted in energy.

Matter-based dogma represents the diminishment of a far greater whole-ism that includes our very perception of self. It suggests that we're living only half a life that is matter dominant. We've opted out on the energetic aspect of our "whole" story. The complete story of our lives is a whole-istic existence that's composed of both matter and energy. Energy based whole-ism is the way of superconscious healing.

Superconscious healing presupposes that every living organism represents a whole comprised of the sum of its parts. True whole-ism is clearly depicted in the greater hierarchy that sequences from energy to matter:

1. Fields

2. Strings

3. Particles

4. Atoms

5. DNA

6. Molecules

7. Cells

8. Tissues

9. Organs

10. Organisms

11. Environments

12. World

13. Solar System

14. Galaxy

15. Universe

16. Multiverse

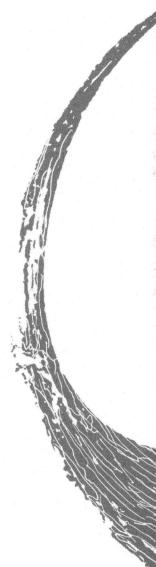

Our current matter-based, mainstream hierarchy begins with cells and omits all energy references that precede the material or cellular life. Superconscious healing posits that our material bias continues to distort our beliefs and limit our healing potential. Everything is energy, and by balancing our various life force energies, we can take a quantum leap in the direction of supporting our superconscious lifestyle.

Together, soul, heart, and loving spirit represent our eternal core self. The material misperception of self is mechanistic, mortal, and ego based. It reflects a mistaken identity.

In order to engage in superconscious healing, we must transform our self-empowerment potential; we must redefine "self," for "self" is the turbine that generates core power. Regarding our limiting perception of self, we need to break down the walls of illusion.

In the Western world, self is an egocentric, willpower-driven concept that aligns with the prevailing ethos. Basically, we're part of a materialistic cultural experiment that has been taught to identify ego as the definition of self.

Because we've been culturally educated from a cellular and not a soul-ular perspective, we've been led to believe that our greatest source of personal power is our will. We live by the credo "If we want something badly enough, we simply have to fight for it." But willpower can only advance intention so far before it begins to deplete more energy than it provides. We can't win all the time. Loss has a way of resulting in self-destruction, which underscores the fact that willpower is not only limited—it's also ultimately disempowering.

All forms of material power are fleeting. Thus, mortality represents the ultimate limitation. The only true, limitless manifestations of transcendent power reside in domains of the immortal. Our only true limitless manifestation of transcendent power resides in the immortal domain of the soul.

To Flow from Source

Soul is arguably the most important and least understood word in any language. I once began a series of seminars by asking the hundreds in attendance for a show of hands from those who believed that the word *soul* was one of the top five most important words in the dictionary. The show of hands was never less than 90 percent. I followed with questions like: Where is your soul? What shape is it? What color is it? What is the purpose of your soul? The awkward responses revealed a distinct disparity. In fact, there's often a decided unease at the mere mention of the word.

Soul, heart, and loving spirit represent the principal elements of our source. Source is not a singular anatomical vessel, nor is it our etheric innards, like a kidney, lung, or liver. We don't possess a source, but we can emanate from source. What we have or don't have is the power of source consciousness, awareness beyond material illusion that leads us to the true nature of our eternal being-ness. Source affords us open access to the highest levels of superconsciousness.

Self represents complex multi-personality divergency that's profoundly mutable and complex. We are forever reacting to the fluctuation of life by consciously and unconsciously shifting from one manifestation of self to another. One minute we recoil from a preoccupation with ego; the next minute we emerge from the luminous radiance of source. Every self is a microcosmic Universe, and the number of expressions of one's self is incalculable. We each elicit a variety of abhorrent, ordinary, extraordinary, and beyond ordinary selves. The goal to achieve a superconscious life of miracles is to avoid slipping into unconscious projections of abhorrent self. Conscious channeling through source is crucial to the prospect of living a life of miracles because we can't expect to actualize the extraordinary by projecting through our ordinary self. Miracles are beyond extraordinary and only source possesses the power to manifest them.

Source awareness represents the awakening moment that we've traveled through endless time and space and died a thousand deaths to give birth to. The mere mention of the word *source* conjures up reflections of all that is profoundly deep and meaningful. The image stirred by the concept of source consciousness crests like beaming swells of radiant light.

Source is a Divine reflection of self as the pure light of consciousness—a light that brandishes the power to transform the mundane into the majestic.

Even as our physical self journeys through the mortal mazes of karmic lessons, source remains a patient promise that is devoted to the destiny of our sacred dharmic liberation. The presence and the power of source serves as a reminder that we've been blessed with the promise of superconsciousness, a promise that enables us to sustain our connection to the divine throughout our never-ending soul's journey. We are immortal beings in a perpetual state of transition.

Change is inevitable; growth is a choice. Only those who consciously invoke change on purpose and resolutely enter the celestial window to the God-mind will become the celebrated purveyors of superconscious miracles.

To Expand the Mind

Generally, we believe that we are ordinary people leading ordinary lives, but we fail to understand and/or accept the potential of the extraordinary nature of self. The concept of extraordinary self should be the focus of our reality.

What percentage of extraordinary potential of your body, mind, and spirit do you believe you're tapped into? What percentage of your extraordinary potential do you believe you have access to at any given moment? What do you think are the most important stimuli to reach your extraordinary potential?

Chances are that your criteria are of a material nature: how much you earn, how much you own, how many friends you have, etc. What if you were to change your criteria from a matter-based to an energy-based standpoint? What if you were to substitute questions like: How powerful is your energy? Do you believe that your energy reflects unlimited potential?

To become superconscious makers of miracles, we might first consider expanding our reality baseline from matter to matter *and* energy. Reality is reliant upon perception and assigned values. The mechanical perception of reality is reliant upon Newtonian physics and solely based on a world of solid objects. It represents a finite view of reality that exists in a universe composed of "thump on it" material objects. Quantum mechanics introduced us to the very smallest scale of energy that reflects an unseen world of infinite possibility based on waves, particles, and atoms.

Quantum mechanics radically altered a fading Newtonian take on reality. It systematically deconstructed previous perceptions about what's real. Through it we have learned that the world isn't made of "stuff" and that the Universe is more like a living organism composed of energy. In this broader reality, each one of us is an integral part of this Universe and what we consciously think profoundly affects its entirety.

Quantum mechanics presents us with a reality that is composed of waves of information that are altered by individual conscious observation. The mere act of paying conscious attention to something not only affects the observed and the observer; it affects all reality. This integral mosaic serves as a reminder that we are part of a greater whole that shares its unlimited powers. We are all part of an infinite field of quantum entanglement. We are in a superposition of multiple possibilities where everything collapses into one-ness and our energy can be present in up to three thousand locations at one time. Quantum mechanics further challenges us with a discourse on the potential power of emptiness.

Everything in the universe is composed of atoms. Atoms are empty, but anything that small that is empty creates a powerful vacuum. If the vacuum of an atom is indeed that powerful, then how could it possibly be empty? An even more compelling question might be: Is the vacuum of the atom filled with nothing or filled with everything? Many experts now presume

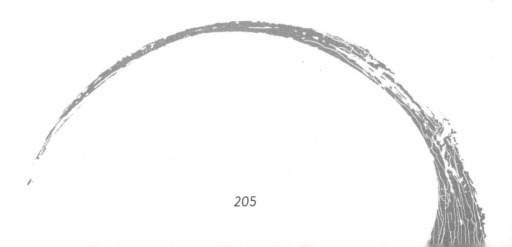

the answer is both. The essence that fills the quantum vacuum of the atom is theorized to be proto-consciousness or pure awareness.

The vacuum in a single hydrogen atom has the equivalent of one trillion times the energy of all the stars and planets in the universe. Each human is composed of 18 billion, billion, billion hydrogen atoms. Based on the limitless potential of our energetic properties, we are truly extraordinary beings that possess capabilities beyond the extraordinary. We are an infinite field of untapped quantum potential that is composed of pure consciousness.

Science is just beginning to understand that the greatest manifestation of power in the Universe is, in fact, proto-consciousness. Imagine, pure awareness is the all-powerful energy that generates the infinite power within the vacuum of every atom. This salient point places us at the threshold of the superconsciousness matter.

If unlimited power is readily attainable, the natural question is: How can we access and, perhaps, even amplify such power? This is a power that manifests as alpha/delta/theta/gamma-burst brain waves, which means we only need to create those brain wave states to catch a glimpse of our superconsciousness. But the process is as much about what we don't do as it is about what we do. We spend so much time in the beta brain-wave state (stressful doing) that it's virtually impossible to get any traction with superconscious power. The more we reformat our mind and brain to live in states of being, as opposed to doing, the more likely we'll be to access and harness this miracle-making state.

Exercise to Flow from Source

For the following Flow from Source exercise, I advise you to record the monologue on your smartphone or other device so that you can play it back as you look into your eyes in the mirror.

Source flows into the soul. Stand before a mirror and focus on the center of your pupils as you recite what I call "The Soul's Invocation." As you listen to the words, believe, from the deepest point of your core, that your soul source is lovingly connecting with you.

"I am who you are. Throughout your eternity of lessons and blessings, I have always been within you and forever so shall remain. I am forever silently observing and assisting you. I remain within you even when you think you're alone. My love for you is unconditional, and I will remain here for you anytime you need me. I am your source of infinite light, Divine inspiration, and Universal transcendence. It is I who makes you the miracle maker you are. Anytime you desire to reach beyond your mortal grasp, I will be here to empower you. I'd like to remind you that you are always far greater and far more powerful than any of your mortal challenges. There is nothing in this world that you cannot overcome. You are immortal. I am the eyes and voice of your soul. We are one, for I am in you as you are in me. Go now and know that you have been blessed to perform miracles. Remember, you need only believe in your own soul."

Afterword

There is a way of miracles. It's achieved through a state of higher consciousness; a consciousness that profoundly inspires our thinking, doing, and being.

An increasing number of people are concluding that it is in their best interest to discover their miracle-making potential. Many are finding themselves drawn to the infinite potential of their transpersonal nature that projects a conscious, positive, proactive self, rather than an unconscious, negative, reactive self. It is also our transpersonal self that extends the presence of higher consciousness to reach beyond accepted limitations with greater expectations. Here, we can extend our powers far beyond momentary states of awareness and can cultivate the long-lasting effects of higher consciousness. In this perpetual state we can exist in uninterrupted meditation and prayer while simultaneously living life. In so doing, we access the unshackled miracle-making power and unlimited healing that we each possess.

Ultimately, the potential of our miracle-making power begins and ends with superconsciousness, which is representative of the unification of our human mind with the mind of God. We do this by shedding the physical world's manipulated illusion of reality that obstructs our miracle-making divine identity. By dedicating ourselves to our higher spiritual presence, prayer, meditation, and evolving self-awareness, we are able to merge our consciousness with the God consciousness. This practice clears the path to overcome the very real, physical, human limitations that prevent us from acknowledging and fully knowing the way of miracles.

In the truest sense, the way of miracles represents an awakening of the divine Source that is our true eternal self. The awakening of the Source within us cultivates an endless stream of superconsciousness that positively affects every aspect of our being. The realization of a divine self within and around us, one that knows no limits, means that we can each choose to be a maker of miracles.

Acknowledgments

My heartfelt thanks to Brit Elders for her tireless support, guidance, and creative brilliance; Devra Jacobs for being the best damn literary agent on the planet; Michele Ashtiani Cohn and Richard Cohn for their belief, trust, and vision; Monique Miller-McCarthy for her superior illustrations; and Fabiola Roht for her countless proofreads.

Glossary

Akashic records: An unwritten record of all human events, thoughts, words, emotions, and intentions that have ever occurred in the past, present, or future

anterior cingulate cortex: A part of the brain that produces the same neurobiological reaction to a real or an imagined event

atman: Sanskrit for the ultimate true self: Our "god" self

astral plane: A nonphysical plane of existence postulated by classical, medieval, oriental, and esoteric philosophies

being-ness: Conscious presence; synonym for *is-ness*

circinate consciousness: The awareness of internal and external existence

Divine "I am": The God-self or soul

Divine mind: The highest attainable consciousness

dharma: The ultimate blessing from righteous living; also known as good *karma*

dis-ease or dis-easing: Illnesses that are created by imbalance in the mind, body, or spirit

ethos: The spirit of a culture

everything-ness: Universal interconnectedness

God-self: The highest manifestation of self

golden calf: Taken from the Old Testament, it represents the idol of materialism that we are obsessively drawn to

half-ness: The absence of wholeness; not being in harmonious balance with the spiritual and physical worlds

heart intelligence: Our emotional IQ

human being-ness: The cultivation of consciousness; more "being," less "doing" in life

human doing-ness: The absence of consciousness; more "doing," less "being" in life

hypnoid dreaming: Daydreaming while hypnotized

hypnagogia: Hallucinations that occur just prior to sleep

hypnopompia: A state of hallucination that occurs when exiting sleep

infinite present: Cultivating a life that's fully conscious and striving for permanence in the moment

is-ness: The conscious presence; synonym for *being-ness*

jagrat: Heightened alertness in a waking state of consciousness

karma: From the Sanskrit word that means "action" or "deed"; generally viewed as lessons that stem from unrighteous living; the opposite of *dharma*

light body: The energy based biofield emitting from the physical body

liminal consciousness: That state of awareness where we've crossed over the threshold of everyday awareness into higher mind

lucid stillness: A meditative-like state

moksha: The total liberation from pain and suffering; the result of *dharma*

mortal "I am": The ego-based personality

nanobe: A bacterium that is the smallest life form currently known to science

neurobiological retention: A resistant stress state where the body, mind, and spirit lose their ability to interconnect and flow

nothing-ness: The absence of presence

panpsychism: Experiences of mental phenomena that are beyond the scope of normal physical explanation; the view that all things, even inanimate, have consciousness

peak living: Living a whole and deeply purposeful life

perspective: A particular attitude toward or a way of regarding something; a point of view

plenary consciousness: Absolute knowingness

presence: Something that exists or is present in a place but is not seen, such as energy

psychosoma: The mental and physical organism as it functions as a cohesive unit, such as how thought or fear can manifest illness by thinking it into existence

qualia: Subjective conscious experiences; the word is derived from the Latin word *qualis*, meaning "what kind of" or "what sort"

self-contempt: Self-separation and self-loathing; what I refer to as original sin

self-transcendence: Rising above your mortal self

sine wave patterns: Oscillating waves produced by energy; a curve or wave representing periodic oscillations of constant amplitude

soul imprinting: The development of awareness of our true soul identity

spiritual mood shifts: The ever-changing states of our deeper awareness

superconscious soul parent: Our innermost spiritual guide

trance manifest: The act of manifesting through trance states

transpectancy: The expectancy of reaching a transformative state

transpersonal: Emanating or going beyond the personal self; concerned especially with esoteric mental experience, such as an altered state of consciousness beyond the usual limits of ego and personality

transmutation: Changing our state of being in such a way that we emanate from source

undivided presence: The act of being completely undistracted and aware

visual creation: A clear imagined vision within the mind

Wuxi: A powerful meditation

yinias: Spiritual energies

Notes

CHAPTER 2

1. Herbert Benson, John W. Lehmann, M. S. Malhotra, Ralph F. Goldman, Jeffrey Hopkins, Mark D. Epstein, "Body Temperature Changes During the Practice of g Tum-mo Yoga," *Nature* 295 (1982): 234–36, https://doi.org/10.1038/295234a0.

2. Center for Cosmology and Astroparticle Physics, Ohio State University, "Humans Really Are Made of Stardust," January 19, 2017, https://ccapp.osu.edu/news/humans-really-are-made-stardust.

3. Robert Rosenthal and Lenore Jacobson, "Teachers' Expectancies: Determinants of Pupils' IQ Gains," *Psychological Reports* 19, no. 1 (1966): 115–18, https://doi.org/10.2466/pr0.1966.19.1.115.

4. Wayne W. Dyer, *You'll See It When You Believe It: The Way to Your Personal Transformation* (New York: Quill, 2001), 49.

5. A. J. Adams, "Your Best Life: From the Comfort of Your Armchair," *Psychology Today*, December 3, 2009, https://www.psychologytoday.com/us/blog/flourish/200912/seeing-is-believing-the-power-visualization.

6. Vinoth K. Ranganathan, Vlodek Siemionow, Jing Z. Liu, Vinod Sahgal, Guang H. Yue, "From Mental Power to Muscle Power by Using the Strength of the Mind," *Neuropsycholigia* 42, no. 7 (2004): 944–56, https://doi.org/10.1016/j.neuropsychologia.2003.11.018.

7. Adyashanti, *The End of Your World: Uncensored Straight Talk on the Nature of Enlightenment* (Boulder, CO: Sounds True, 2008), 136–137.

CHAPTER 3

1. Eknath Easwaran, *The Upanishads: A Classic of Indian Spirituality*, 2nd ed. (Marin County, CA: Nilgiri Press, 2007).

2. Carl G. Jung, *The Undiscovered Self* (Boston: Little Brown, 1958).

3. Christopher C. Davoli and Richard A. Abrams, "Reaching Out With the Imagination," *Psychological Science* 20, no. 3 (March 1, 2009), 293–95, https://journals.sagepub.com /doi/10.1111/j.1467-9280.2009.02293.x.
4. Paul Twitchell, *Eckankar, The Key to Secret Worlds*, 1st ed. (Chanhassen, MN: Eckankar, 1969).
5. Paul P. Pearsall, PhD, *The Heart's Code* (New York: Broadway Books, 1998).
6. John A. Armour, "Anatomy and Function of the Intrathoracic Neurons Regulating the Mammalian Heart," in *Reflex Control of the Circulation*, eds. Irving H. Zucker and Joseph P. Gilmore (Boca Raton, FL: CRC Press, 1991).
7. "Interconnectivity Tree Research Project," HeartMath Institute website, June 29, 2016, https://www.heartmath.org/calendar-of-events /interconnectivity-tree-research-project/.
8. Elizabeth B. Raposa, Holly B. Laws, and Emily B. Ansell, "Prosocial Behavior Mitigates the Negative Effects of Stress in Everyday Life," *Clinical Psychological Science* 4, no. 4 (December 10, 2015), 691–98, https://doi.org/10.1177/2167702615611073.
9. Mark Mincolla, PhD, *Whole Health: A Holistic Approach to Healing for the 21st Century* (New York: TarcherPerigee, 2013), 245.
10. Herbert Benson, John W. Lehmann, M. S. Malhotra, Ralph F. Goldman, Jeffrey Hopkins, and Mark D. Epstein, "Body Temperature Changes During the Practice of g Tum-mo Yoga," Nature 295 (1982), 234–36, https://doi.org/10.1038/295234a0.
11. Alan S. Cowen and Dacher Keltner, *Self-report Captures 27 Distinct Categories of Emotion Bridged by Continuous Gradients* (University of California at Berkeley: Proceedings of the National Academy of Sciences, 2017).
12. Sigmund Freud, *Beyond the Pleasure Principle* (New York: W.W. Norton, 1990).

CHAPTER 4

1. Hans Selye, *The Stress of Life* (New York: McGraw-Hill, 1956).
2. "Heart Disease Facts," Centers for Disease Control and Prevention, last modified September 8, 2020, https://www.cdc.gov/heartdisease/facts.htm#:~:text=Heart% 20Disease%20in%20the%20United%20States&text=About%20655%2C000%20 Americans%20die%20from,1%20in%20every%204%20deaths.&text=Heart% 20disease%20costs%20the%20United,year%20from%202014%20to%202015.&text =This%20includes%20the%20cost%20of,lost%20productivity%20due%20to %20death.
3. The American Cancer Society, "Cancer Facts and Figures 2019," The American Cancer Society website, accessed January 12, 2021, https://www.cancer.org/content/dam /cancer-org/research/cancer-facts-and-statistics/annual-cancer-facts-and-figures/2019 /cancer-facts-and-figures-2019.pdf
4. Roma Pahwa, Amandeep Goyal, Pankaj Bansal, and Ishwarlal Jialal, "Chronic Inflammation," StatPearls website, last updated November 20, 2020, https://www.ncbi .nlm.nih.gov/books/NBK493173/.
5. Renee Morad, "How Diet Can Change Your DNA: Recent Studies Suggest That the Food You Eat Could Modify Your Genes and Potentially Your Children's," *Scientific*

American, June 7, 2017, https://www.scientificamerican.com/custom-media/science
-for-life/how-diet-can-change-your-dna/.

6. Marta Crous-Bou, Teresa T. Fung, Jennifer Prescott, Bettina Julin, Mengmeng Du, Qi
Sun, Kathryn M. Rexrode, Frank B. Hu, and Immaculata De Vivo, "Mediterranean
Diet and Telomere Length in Nurses' Health Study: Population Based Cohort Study,"
BMJ 2014, no. 349 (December 2, 2014): g6674, https://doi.org/10.1136/bmj.g6674.

7. Eli Puterman, Jue Lin, Elizabeth Blackburn, Aoife O'Donovan, Nancy Adler, and
Elissa Epel, "The Power of Exercise: Buffering the Effect of Chronic Stress on
Telomere Length," *PLoS One* 7, no. 5 (May 26, 2010), https://doi.org/10.1371/journal.
pone.0010837.

8. Vicki Brower, "Mind-body Research Moves Towards the Mainstream," *EMBO Reports*,
April 1, 2006, https://doi.org/10.1038/sj.embor.7400671.

9. Esther M. Sternberg, "Walter B. Cannon and '"Voodoo" Death': A Perspective from 60
Years On," *American Journal of Public Health* 92, no. 10 (October 2002): 1564–1566,
https://doi.org/10.2105/AJPH.92.10.1564.

10. Rachel Zelkowitz, "The Placebo Effect: Not All in Your Head," *Science*, December 2,
2008, https://www.sciencemag.org/news/2008
/12/placebo-effect-not-all-your-head.

CHAPTER 6

1. Adrian Cho, "Quantum Experiment in Space Confirms That Reality Is What You
Make It," *Science*, October 27, 2017, https://www.sciencemag.org/news/2017/10/
quantum
-experiment-space-confirms-reality-what-you-make-it-0.

2. Albert Maslow, quoted in M. A. Carrano, *Asleep in the Helix: Survival and the Science of
Self-Realization* (North Haven, CT: Avatar Paradigms, 2009), 270.

3. Mario Orsatti, "New Study Sheds Light on 'Peak Experiences' in World-Class
Performers," *TM Blog*, Transcendental Meditation, August 24, 2012, https://www
.tm.org/blog/students/study-on-peak
-experiences/.

CHAPTER 7

1. Mark Mincolla, *Whole Health Diet* (New York: TarcherPerigree, 2015), 262.

2. "Food Additives," Food Safety Education, The University of Rhode Island, last
modified accessed January 12, 2021, https://web.uri.edu/foodsafety/food-additives/.

3. Euridice Martinez Steele, Larissa Galastri Baraldi, Maria Laura da Costa Louzada,
Jean-Claude Moubarac, Dariush Mozaffarian, and Carlos Augusto Monteiro, "Ultra-
Processed Foods and Added Sugars in the US Diet: Evidence from a Nationally
Representative Cross-Sectional Study," *BMJ Open*, 6 (2016): e009892, http://dx.doi
.org/10.1136/bmjopen-2015-009892.

4. Ruchi S. Gupta, Christopher M. Warren, Bridget M. Smith, Jialing Jiang, Jesse
A. Blumenstock, Matthew M. Davis, Robert P. Schleimer, and Kari C. Nadeau,

"Prevalence and Severity of Food Allergies Among US Adults," *Jama Network Open* 2, no. 1 (2019): e185630, doi:10.1001/jamanetworkopen.2018.5630.

CHAPTER 8
1. Derek Beres, "Psilocybin 'Markedly' Boosts Feelings of Self-Transcendence During Meditation," *Big Think*, October 28, 2019, https://bigthink.com/personal-growth/psilocybin-meditation.
2. Melody Petersen, *Our Daily Meds* (New York: Sarah Crichton Books, 2008), 7.

Recommended Reading

*The Biology of Belief: Unleashing the Power of Consciousness, Matter &
Miracles* by Bruce H. Lipton (Hay House, Inc., 2016)

Healing Ourselves: Biofield Science and the Future of Health by Shamini
Jain, PhD (Sounds True, 2021)

Heart Intelligence: Connecting with the Intuitive Guidance of the Heart by
Doc Childre, Howard Martin, Deborah Rozman, and Rollin McCraty
(Waterfront Digital Press, 2016)

The Heart's Code: Tapping the Wisdom and Power of Our Heart Energy by
Paul Pearsall, PhD (Broadway Books, NY, 1999)

Metahuman: Unleashing Your Infinite Potential by Deepak Chopra, MD
(Penguin RandomHouse, 2019)

Morphic Resonance: The Nature of Formative Causation by Rupert
Sheldrake (Inner Traditions/Bear & Co., 2009)

Whole Health: A Holistic Approach to Healing for the 21st Century by Mark
Mincolla, PhD (TarcherPerigee, 2013)

The Whole Health Diet: A Transformational Approach to Weight Loss by
Mark Mincolla, PhD (TarcherPerigee, 2015)